Contemporary Public Health

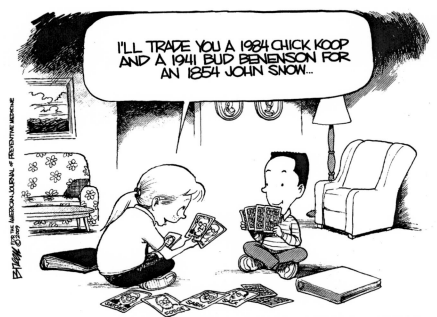

IF PUBLIC HEALTH WERE AS POPULAR AS OUR NATIONAL PASTIME

CONTEMPORARY PUBLIC HEALTH

Principles, Practice, and Policy

Edited by
James W. Holsinger Jr.

Foreword by
David M. Lawrence

Emmanuel D. Jadhav
Assistant to the Editor

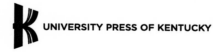

UNIVERSITY PRESS OF KENTUCKY

Scholarly publisher for the Commonwealth,
serving Bellarmine University, Berea College, Centre College of Kentucky,
Eastern Kentucky University, The Filson Historical Society, Georgetown
College, Kentucky Historical Society, Kentucky State University, Morehead State
University, Murray State University, Northern Kentucky University, Transylvania
University, University of Kentucky, University of Louisville, and Western
Kentucky University.

Editorial and Sales Offices: The University Press of Kentucky
663 South Limestone Street, Lexington, Kentucky 40508-4008
www.kentuckypress.com

Frontispiece © 2010 *American Journal of Preventive Medicine.* Concept by
Charlotte Seidman to honor Abram S. Benenson and all the pioneers of public
health and preventive medicine, and executed by Steve Breen, Pulitzer Prize–
winning political cartoonist for the *San Diego Union-Tribune.*

17 16 15 14 13   5 4 3 2 1

Library of Congress Cataloging-in-Publication Data

Contemporary public health : principles, practice, and policy / edited by James
W. Holsinger Jr. ; foreword by David M. Lawrence.
    p. ; cm.
  Includes bibliographical references and index.
  ISBN 978-0-8131-4123-7 (hardcover : alk. paper) —
  ISBN 978-0-8131-4125-1 (epub) — ISBN 978-0-8131-4124-4 (pdf)
  I. Holsinger, James W.
  [DNLM: 1. Delivery of Health Care—United States—Essays. 2. Public
Health—United States—Essays. 3. Health Policy—United States—Essays. WA 9]
    362.10973—dc23   201202958

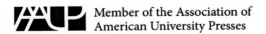 Member of the Association of
American University Presses

Contents

Dedication

F. Douglas Scutchfield, MD

F. Douglas Scutchfield was born and reared in Eastern Kentucky. His early years in Appalachia have had a lasting influence on his life and work, resulting in a lifelong passion for the health of Kentuckians and medically underserved Americans. He graduated with distinction from Eastern Kentucky University in 1962, where he met and married Phyllis and where he received an honorary doctor of science degree in 2004. Scutch graduated from the University of Kentucky College of Medicine in 1966 at age twenty-three and was elected a member of Alpha Omega Alpha. During the next four years, he completed a rotating internship at Northwestern Medical Center in Chicago, a fellowship as an epidemic intelligence service officer at the Centers for Disease Control and Prevention, and a preventive medicine residency at the University of Kentucky Chandler Medical Center.

Recruited to Morehead, Kentucky, to practice family medicine, he was a charter diplomate of the American Board of Family Practice. While practicing in Morehead, he received faculty appointments to the University of Kentucky, the University of Louisville, and Morehead State University, and he established the first hospital-based home health service in Kentucky. His mentor, Dr. William R. Willard, vice president for health affairs and founding dean of the University of Kentucky College of Medicine, recruited him to the University of Alabama, where Scutch served as professor and chair of the Department of Family Medicine and Community Medicine for the next five years and, subsequently, associate dean for academic affairs in the College of Community Health Sciences.

Scutch's education in public health and prevention established his career-long love for community and population health issues and policy, including assessing the need for public health services and developing public health systems policy. His early interest in the socioecological determinants of health quickly became apparent in his publications, as did his nascent interest in public health services and systems research, an area that he would create virtually single-handedly in the years to come. His thinking developed around the role of community-oriented primary care as a means of improving health care for the underserved.

In 1979 Scutch was asked to become the first director of the Graduate School of Public Health at San Diego State University. There, his interest in the education of the public health workforce grew rapidly, along with his participation in the publication of a variety of professional and academic journals. He served as editor in chief, editor, or member of the editorial board of several medical journals, but most importantly, the *American Journal of Preventive Medicine.* His collaboration with C. William Keck, MD, culminated in the writing of *Principles of Public Health Practice,* a premier public health textbook.

In 1997 Scutch returned to the University of Kentucky to become the founding director of the School of Public Health. At the pinnacle of his career, he has played a key role in the development of public health accreditation and quality improvement over the last fifteen years, serving as a founding member of the Public Health Accrediting Board. In association with the Robert Wood Johnson Foundation and the Centers for Disease Control and Prevention, he has led two national programs of excellence, the Center for Public Health Services and Systems Research and the Center of Excellence for Public Health Workforce Research and Policy, and he recently created the National Coordinating Center for Public Health Services and Systems Research.

During a sabbatical at the Kettering Foundation, Scutch's interest was sparked by the concept of making democracy work in the public sector of community health. His long-standing effort to involve governmental and nongovernmental organizations in public health was an outgrowth of his efforts to engage the public in their own health care. While Dozor visiting professor at Ben Gurion University of the Negev in Israel, he expanded his public health interests internationally.

In addition to his writing and academic pursuits, Scutch has been significantly involved in American medicine at the local, state, and national levels. As a result of his longtime service to the American Medical Association, he received both the William Beaumont Award and the association's Distinguished Service Award. A fellow of the American College of Preventive Medicine, he served as its president from 1989 to 1991. In 1992 he received its Distinguished Service Award and in 1999 its Special Recognition Award. After being elected president of the Association of Teachers of Preventive Medicine (1981–1982), he was awarded the Duncan Clark Award. He is currently a member of the Board of Regents of the National Library of Medicine.

Throughout his career, Scutch has created and actively maintained an extensive network of friends consisting of former students, fellow faculty members, staff members, and professional colleagues. He is a man of few acquaintances but a multitude of friends, whom he serves with abandon. A man of deep tenderness, despite his size, he cares deeply for and about the people in his life. Because of his role as a doctor's doctor and a public health practitioner's practitioner, and in honor of his lifetime of service to the profession of medicine and, specifically, to the area of community and public health, Dr. F. Douglas Scutchfield's friends and colleagues dedicate this book to him.

James W. Holsinger Jr., MD, PhD
April 23, 2012

Foreword

Years ago, during a sabbatical from the School of Public Health he founded at San Diego State University, Doug Scutchfield joined our family for dinner one evening. At the time, our children were of an age when they considered adults to be uninformed and uninteresting. Listening to old fogies tell war stories was not high on their lists of favorite things to do. But as Doug related tale after tale about our medical school experiences, the children sat enthralled long after dinner was finished and the last plate had been cleared. At the end of each story, they joined my wife and me in helpless laughter and then pleaded for "one more. Tell us another."

That is how most of us feel about Scutch. Give us more. Take on one more challenge in public health. Help us learn and laugh together. In his dedication, Jim Holsinger describes Scutch's remarkable career: the impact he has had on his chosen field and the many people with whom he has come in contact as teacher, colleague, and friend. I count myself fortunate to be a lifetime colleague and a friend since that first day in medical school a half century ago. And, like Dr. Holsinger and the many others who have contributed to this volume, I am honored to be a part of this expression of gratitude to Scutch for his contributions to our field and our lives.

This can be nothing other than an ambitious book, given the person we honor. The subjects it covers range widely across the history, current issues, and future challenges in public health. As only the best of essays can, this collection stimulates and provokes. The authors offer the reader the gift of perspective, which is often missing in the classic text format. These essays are intended to supplement formal texts, round out a subject, introduce context and nuance, and provide insights into the thinking of seasoned practitioners. The volume benefits from the care with which each essay has been crafted, the guidance provided by Jim Holsinger, and the editing by the team at the University Press of Kentucky. It more than realizes its ambitions to teach and to honor.

It also comes at an important time. Around the globe, in country after country, we confront the limits of the traditional medical model. It is expensive and contributes only marginally to the health of our communities. We don't get what we pay for in terms of better health, better quality of lives, or better personal and workforce productivity. As the essays in this collection demonstrate, this is where public health can play a crucial role.

The field's rich history and modern advances have contributed to the health of communities in countless ways throughout the world. Now, by focusing on community and population health, adapting the ubiquitous technologies of the Internet and mobile telephony, building the capacity to manage complex data analytics, and continuing to push the boundaries of population and molecular science, public health holds great promise that it can provide better health care at lower costs than we have achieved through our long infatuation with and stunning investments in the medical model. If we can wrestle to the ground the issues of organization and funding that have plagued the field of public health for at least two centuries, we have a shot at making a major difference. At no time has doing so been more important.

To Scutch, friend and colleague, thank you for providing the impetus to write this important book. It does you proud, I believe. It is a fitting tribute to someone who has advanced the field so tirelessly and unselfishly for so many years.

David M. Lawrence, MD, MPH
Chairman and CEO (retired)
Kaiser Foundation Health Plan and Hospitals Inc.

Preface

The practice of public health has traveled a long and often storied path. In the United States this path has often been rocky, causing progress to come in fits and starts. Historically, the education of public health practitioners has been the purview of the various professional disciplines engaged in its practice: medicine, nursing, sanitation (environmental health), biostatistics, laboratory science, management. The Welch-Rose report of 1915 paved the way to separate the education of public health practitioners from that of physicians. As a result, the first school of public health was founded at Johns Hopkins University in 1916, and by the mid-1940s, schools of public health were being accredited. For a number of years a core group of twenty-three schools or colleges of public health existed to serve the educational needs of the profession. By the end of the twentieth century and into the early years of the twenty-first, the number of public health academic programs exploded. Consequently, the number of students enrolled in master's and doctor of public health programs has grown at a rapid pace. Although it consists of a number of separate and long-standing academic disciplines, public health as an academic discipline in its own right is relatively recent. As a result, the number of textbooks related to public health as a discipline has grown in an effort to serve this expanding body of students.

How does *Contemporary Public Health* intersect with this educational venture? This text is composed of essays commissioned specifically to elaborate on the material found in traditional public health practice textbooks. The essays are designed to accompany introductory courses in public health practice at the graduate level, although they may be of assistance in upper-division undergraduate courses as well. The essays may also serve practitioners who are engaged in continuing their education, either individually or collectively in various venues. The authors provide both public health students and practitioners alike with a contemporary picture of public health in the early twenty-first century. The goal of the book is to encourage current and future practitioners to serve their communities with a clearer understanding of the trajectory of American public health today.

Acknowledgments are due to a number of individuals who assisted in the development of this book. The editorial assistance of Rebecca S. Friend was, as usual, exceptional. Her patience in dealing with the intricacies of a multiauthor project proved invaluable. Emmanuel D. Jadhav, a doctoral student and graduate assistant, exhibited never-failing good humor, even in the midst of sorting out two separate but contiguous writing projects. Stephen M. Wrinn, director of the University Press of Kentucky and acquisitions editor for this project, was a constant companion along the way. His friendship and support never wavered, and I am in his debt. I am grateful to my colleagues who wrote the essays included herein for taking the time from their busy lives to honor Dr. F. Douglas Scutchfield, an exceptional friend. They were more than gracious in receiving my many cajoling e-mails, and I deeply appreciate their encouragement and support. My wife, Dr. Barbara Craig Holsinger, read, reviewed, and corrected significant portions of the book and, as usual during such projects, lived with a husband whose mind was often elsewhere, regardless of where his body was located physically. She is a pearl without price!

James W. Holsinger Jr., MD, PhD

Introduction

History and Context of Public Health Care

James W. Holsinger Jr. and F. Douglas Scutchfield

The history of public health in the United States demonstrates cycles of action and inaction, funding and a lack thereof. From its inception in 1798 until the post–September 11, 2001, period, the development of public health, according to Fee and Brown, has been "consistently plagued by organizational inefficiencies, jurisdictional irrationalities, and chronic underfunding. It is apparent that public health—in addition to lacking the support it deserves—has long been subject to a social and cultural discounting, especially in comparison to high-technology medicine, which undermines its authority."[1] A review of its history results in understanding that public health is favored politically and fiscally during and immediately after periods of crisis, only to slip into obscurity once the crisis has passed. The result of such attention and inattention is the lack of a clear trajectory in providing for the health of the American population and its communities.

Seaport Epidemics and the First Boards of Health

On July 16, 1798, President John Adams signed an act passed by the Fifth Congress of the United States that provided for "the temporary relief and maintenance of sick or disabled seamen in the hospitals or other proper institutions now established in the several ports of the United States, or in ports where no such institutions exist, then in such other manner as he [the secretary of the treasury] shall direct."[2] The act was a response to epidemic diseases such as smallpox, typhoid fever, plague, and especially yellow fever that were ravaging the eastern seaports. Notions of public health were rudimentary at best, with quarantine being one of the most effective mechanisms for dealing with outbreaks of epidemics, which were often thought to be initiated by seamen returning from lengthy voyages to foreign lands. These returning merchant seamen, who were often ill and lacked family at their ports of debarkation, were a burden on seaport communities, and the need to care for them resulted in the creation of the Marine Hospital Service. This new system also assured healthier merchant mariners for the nation's expanding commercial ventures.

In addition to the efforts of the federal government, local and state governments were attempting to protect their populations from the various catastrophic infectious diseases that traumatized port cities, such as the yellow fever epidemic of 1793 in Philadelphia.[3] Although the responses to yellow fever were broad based, they usually involved cities creating boards of health. "From about 1793 to 1806 yellow fever posed a major threat up and down the East Coast and created a heightened consciousness of public health, then understood as the set of measures undertaken to protect the local population from epidemic disease. Philadelphia organized a Board of Health in 1794; Baltimore in 1797; Boston in 1799; Washington, D.C., in 1802; and New Orleans in 1804."[1] In dealing with the public health issue of epidemic diseases, the lack of a clear understanding of the theoretical basis of infectious disease was a major impediment to disease control. For example, during this period, the contagionist and miasmatist theories of public health intervention competed for favor among boards of health. The contagionist theory was based on controlling environmental conditions as well as isolating infected individuals by quarantine. Houses, belongings, and goods were fumigated in an effort to contain the contagion of epidemic disease. The miasmatist theory was based on the development of protective measures against malodorous urban nuisances such as garbage and filth of all kinds, which resulted in garbage removal and street cleaning. Given the local nature of these two theories of the spread of disease, local communities became deeply involved in dealing with epidemic infectious diseases during this period of our nation's history.

The U.S. Constitution does not specifically reserve health as a power of the federal government; therefore, each state bears responsibility for the health of its citizens. As a result, various states enacted legislation authorizing local public health boards to utilize their police powers to enforce quarantines and disinfection measures (contagionist theory) and to undertake garbage removal and street cleaning (miasmatist theory). However, as would happen again and again in the ensuing years, as the threat to the public's health from yellow fever and other infectious diseases diminished, so did the enthusiasm for public health measures. Business leaders were opposed to continuing the practices developed by the local boards because they believed such activities interfered with commercial interests, and many local boards were abolished.

Cholera, Civil War, and Sanitation

A new threat became apparent in the 1830s, a period of urban growth coinciding with the accumulation of waste, including excrement and garbage, and the pollution of community water supplies. These conditions resulted in the spread of epidemic diseases involving waterborne enteric discharges with fecal to oral spread, especially cholera. When New York City was threatened by a cholera outbreak in 1832, its board of health responded with inaction. Business leaders had gained control of the board and accused physicians and others of disrupting the economic life of the city.[4] With cholera rampaging through the city's slums and wealthy citizens fleeing, the board of health was prevented from taking action to contain the epidemic. The result was that "these sudden catastrophic events compelled even politicians and business leaders to devote their attention to sanitary improvements, city cleanliness, quarantine, and hospital expansion."[5] Thus, as cholera spread through the country, voluntary committees and boards of health were reestablished in an effort to fight the epidemic. Other infectious disease epidemics also swept the country during this period, only to be met with indifference by citizens and leaders alike, due to their familiarity with the diseases and a certain sense of helplessness in the face of the calamity. However, as each epidemic abated, "politicians tended to ignore the fate of the multitudes of immigrant poor, unless compelled to action by the insistent demands of reform groups or the fear of popular unrest."[5]

A similar response occurred when the Shattuck report was published in 1850 by the Massachusetts Sanitary Commission. Although viewed as a landmark in the development of community health action, the report had virtually no effect in its own day. Its major recommendation was the creation of a state board of health, which required an additional nineteen years to implement.[6] As a consequence of this inaction, the emphasis on public health was blighted until the next major calamity, which was usually not long in coming.

By the late 1850s, efforts had begun to move public health beyond the control of local city politicians. The American Civil War resulted in the next wave of reform. Consciousness was raised nationally when it became apparent that more soldiers were dying of disease than as a result of enemy action. Nearly 250,000 Union soldiers died of infectious diseases spread by the unsanitary conditions in the military camps. As a result, the sanitary reformers of the period "persuaded President Lincoln to create a Sanitary Commission to investigate conditions besetting the Union forces. The commission pressured both civilian and military authorities to improve sanitation and to educate officers and enlisted men about the spread of infectious diseases and the need for personal and public hygiene."[1] With the Union army's capture of important southern cities, its sanitary program was implemented there and continued after the conclusion of the war. In a very real sense, the Civil War served as a turning point in the history of public health in the United States. One early result of the war and the sanitary movement was the creation of the American Public Health Association (APHA) in 1872 for the express purpose of "the advancement of sanitary science and the promotion of organizations and measures for the practical application of public hygiene."[7] In many ways, this marked the beginning of the modern American public health era.

During the same period, the Marine Hospital Service failed to live up to expectations. It was "not a system in any contemporary sense of the word but, rather, a loose entitlement managed largely by customs, collectors and politicians. Where hospitals were built, they were often crowded or badly staffed and sick seamen were often forced to seek shelter in municipal alms houses. Contract services offered in their stead were frequently unavailable or of poor quality."[8] As is often the case with government facilities, many of the Marine Hospital Service's hospitals were located based on political whim rather than the needs of merchant mariners or the service itself. During the Civil War, Union or Confederate forces utilized many of these facilities as hospitals or barracks, and some were demolished. As a result, by the end of the war, only eight of twenty-seven Marine Hospital Service facilities were operational. "In spite of the criticisms and recommendations, national reform of management of the hospitals was not possible due to the absence of any central concept to the program."[8] In 1869 the entire system was reviewed extensively at the direction of the secretary of the treasury, under whose auspices it functioned. The resulting report again decried the abject nature of the facilities, resulting in federal legislation in 1870 that created the position of supervising surgeon of the Marine Hospital Service. This post was the forerunner of the modern surgeon general of the Public Health Service and constituted a vital and significant change toward improving the system.

Interregnum and the National Board of Health

Between the Civil War and the period of mass immigration to the United States at the turn of the century, a major public health battle was fought and lost. The first supervising surgeon of the Marine Hospital Service, John Maynard Woodworth, revolutionized the service through a variety of reforms, including shepherding the Quarantine Act of 1878 through Congress. The previous federal quarantine law had been inadequate, requiring federal agents to abide by various state laws. Following a yellow fever epidemic in New Orleans that spread rapidly northward throughout the Mississippi Valley, national attention was drawn to the need for a federal quarantine policy. This new legislation gave the Marine Hospital Service quarantine authority for the nation—the first expansion of its mission beyond the care of merchant seamen.

In an attempt to recast the national health agenda, efforts were made to create a National Health Department. Due to internecine conflict among the proponents of such a development, the effort failed. Instead, a National Board of Health was created, but its ability to direct change was sorely constrained by the requirement of congressional reauthorization of its funding after four years. During its existence, the National Board of Health absorbed the national quarantine function of the Marine Hospital Service, thus defeating efforts to expand the service's functions. The board's actions included establishing a national program of public health surveillance and intervention that involved grants to states for sanitary work and publication of the *Bulletin*, the forerunner of *Public Health Reports*, which continues today. "With no further outbreak of yellow fever to frighten Congress into stronger action, the National Board of Health was allowed to expire in 1883, and national responsibility for quarantine and public health, such as it was, reverted back to the Marine Hospital Service."[1] As a consequence, this short-lived period of national public health activity came to an abrupt end.

Immigration and the Birth of Progressivism

At the end of the nineteenth century, a new public health threat appeared on the horizon as "huge waves of immigrants, especially from Eastern and Southern Europe, were now entering the country while harboring (many suspected) all manner of genetic defects and infectious diseases."[1] Many of the nearly 24 million individuals who arrived between 1880 and 1920 immigrated to participate in the growing prosperity of the United States and to meet the need for laborers in the growing industrial sector.[9]

Clearly, public health was in ferment owing to both the increase in immigration and the enormous biological discoveries of the late nineteenth century, including the identification of numerous epidemic-causing infectious agents.[8] The rise in immigration coincided with an outbreak of cholera in eastern Europe and Russia, resulting in the National Quarantine Act of 1893, which enhanced the quarantine role of the Marine Hospital Service. Specifically, the act required that individuals with dangerous contagious diseases be prevented from entering the United States. The Marine Hospital Service therefore surveyed and inspected all local and state quarantine stations, including Ellis Island in New York Harbor, the major point of entry into the United States for large numbers of immigrants. As the service expanded its mission, including the creation of the Hygienic Laboratory, it was renamed the Public Health and Marine Hospital Service in 1902, and by 1912 it had come into its own as the U.S. Public Health Service.

By the turn of the century, public health reform was pressing forward on numerous fronts. The industrial transformation of the nineteenth century had changed the core of the nation. Even though the causes of infectious diseases had been discovered, the "burgeoning health problems of the industrial cities could not be ignored; almost all families lost children to diphtheria, smallpox, or other infectious diseases."[5] Poverty and disease became linked in the minds of many and were seen as the consequence of the nation's urbanization, immigration, and industrialization. Pressure mounted for appropriate responses to the root causes of the social aspects of public health problems, resulting in the development of social reform movements across the country. These social reform groups targeted the social issues of the day as well as working diligently for a variety of social improvements. The practitioners of various professions banded together with health reformers to improve the sanitary conditions of the cities. "The field of public hygiene exemplified a happy marriage of engineers, physicians, and public spirited citizens providing a model of complementary comportment under the banner of sanitary science."[10] Thus, the Progressive Era was born with a renewed sense of purpose and a zeal to deal with the issue of vulnerable individuals in need of assistance.

In the early 1900s a broad spectrum of American citizens engaged in efforts to improve housing, sanitation, occupational safety, maternal and child health, school hygiene, and a variety of significant issues facing the urban poor. "The progressive reform groups in the public health movement advocated immediate change tempered by scientific knowledge and humanitarian concern. Sharing the revolutionaries' perception of the plight of the poor and the injustices of the system, they nonetheless counseled less radical solutions. They advocated public health reforms on political, economic, humanitarian, and scientific grounds. Politically, public health reform offered a middle ground between cutthroat principles of entrepreneurial capitalism and the revolutionary ideas of the socialists, anarchists, and utopian visionaries."[5] During this period, the leaders in public health argued that a cost-benefit analysis of the issues would allow a determination of the most appropriate decisions to be implemented.[11] However, the Progressive movement created controversy with the organization of the Committee of One Hundred for National Health in 1906, whose purpose was to create a national department of health. In some respects, this reprised the fight over the creation of the National Board of Health in 1879. In concept, the goal was to consolidate all federal health agencies, including the Public Health and Marine Hospital Service, into a single department.

By 1920, thirteen bills had been introduced in Congress proposing changes to the Public Health and Marine Hospital Service or the creation of a national health department. The failure to create a national health department resulted in the expansion of the Public Health Service's mission in 1912. The newly renamed organization was empowered, in addition to its efforts to combat the spread of diseases, to investigate not only the pollution of navigable lakes and streams but also their sanitation.[12] "By 1915, the Public Health Service, the United States Army, and the Rockefeller Foundation were the major agencies involved in public health activities, supplemented on a local level by a network of city and state health departments."[5]

In 1910 the Flexner report, on the status of medical education in the United States and Canada, constituted a significant health care response to the Progressive Era.[13] Although the report did not specifically address the educational needs related to public health, it spurred the Welch-Rose report of 1915, which, under the auspices of the Rockefeller Foundation, addressed the requirement for a public health workforce separate from curative-oriented medical practice and the need to develop academic training programs for public health practitioners. Welch's report described and justified the creation of an institute, which he would found a year later as the Johns Hopkins School of Hygiene and Public Health. He had a clear purpose in mind: the "development of the spirit of investigation and the advancement of knowledge" and the provision of "advanced workers and investigators to be teachers, authorities and experts . . . for service in different fields."[14] The Rockefeller Foundation responded to Welch's report by funding his institute—the first formally endowed school of public health in the United States and the beginning of modern public health education. Thus, as the Progressive Era began to wind down, the practice of public health was beginning to professionalize.

Reaction to the Progressive Era

A conservative political reaction followed the Progressive Era. At the same time, World War I began in Europe, and by 1917 the United States had joined the war effort. The war resulted in a number of federal laws, including the Espionage Act of 1917 and the Sedition Act of 1918, which gave the president broad powers to deal with individuals and organizations critical of the U.S. government. By 1920 the Justice Department had summarily deported more than 6,000 aliens.[15] "Quota laws and acts in 1921 and 1924 limited the immigration of each nationality to 2 percent of what it had been in 1890, thus deliberately favoring immigration from northern and western Europe over eastern and southern Europeans."[1] As a result, immigration into the United States effectively came to a standstill.

As the Progressive Era ended, public health began a decline that would last until the health issues of the Great Depression and World War II reinvigorated it. "Between 1920 and 1930 Republicans controlled the White House, the Senate, and the House of Representatives. In this conservative, resurgently free-market era, Progressivism further declined and public health itself came under suspicion."[5] A major conservative reaction occurred within organized medicine, and a battle over the Sheppard-Towner Maternity and Infancy Protection Act of 1921 created a division in the medicine and public health professions. This act "authorized federal grants-in-aid to states to promote the health of mothers and children. The AMA [American Medical Association] and most of its affiliated state societies strongly opposed the measure, asserting that it threatened the American home, invaded states rights, and was completely unnecessary. . . . Although unsuccessful in stopping passage of the Sheppard-Towner Act, organized medicine steadily lobbied against it and managed to prevent its reenactment in 1929."[16] In 1926 the president of the APHA pushed back against the detractors of public health, calling their attacks politically destructive, superficial, and frivolous.[17] This struggle over maternal and child health services and who should deliver them—public health or medicine—created a division that remains a source of concern to both professions.

As twentieth-century public health reformers adopted a narrower and more technical view of their work—in contrast to nineteenth-century reformers' broad interest in the social welfare of their fellow citizens—profound limitations in the scope of public health became evident. The difference between the broad and narrow approaches to public health resulted in an explicit backing away from necessary reforms. To illustrate, as Rosenkrantz points out, a Massachusetts commission dominated by physicians recommended in 1936 that the state abandon even preventive medicine and suggested that "the scope of public health be limited to the regulation of the environment and the provision of technical aid to the physician."[18] Starr summarizes the situation effectively:

> In retrospect, the turn of the century now seems to have been a golden age for public health, when its achievements followed one another in dizzying succession and its future possibilities seemed limitless. By the thirties, the expansionary era had come to an end, and the functions of public health were becoming more fixed and routine. The bacteriological revolution had played itself out in the organization of public services, and soon the introduction of antibiotics and other

drugs would enable private physicians to reclaim some of their functions, like the treatment of venereal disease and tuberculosis. Yet it had been clear, long before, that public health in America was to be "relegated to a secondary status: less prestigious than clinical medicine, less amply financed, and blocked from assuming the higher-level functions of coordination and direction"[1] that might have developed had it not been banished from medical care.[19]

Thus, the field of public health had reached another nadir as its erstwhile allies, physicians, veered away from its support.

The Depression, the New Deal, and World War II

The onset of the Great Depression in 1929 provided a major stimulus for the development of public health practice. Reports by a private commission, the Committee on the Costs of Medical Care, determined that public health was in dire straits: only 3.3 cents of each health care dollar was expended on public health endeavors, a situation not substantially different from today. According to the committee, these "niggardly appropriations not only seriously limit present activities, but also hamper medical schools in their efforts to attract competent students to public health careers."[20] The Depression itself brought the committee's efforts to a halt, and "as banks failed, industrial production dropped, wages fell, and unemployment climbed, state and local health departments found their budgets slashed while the demand for their services soared."[1] Following the election of 1932 and the advent of the New Deal, the Public Health Service became part of a major effort to revitalize the nation economically. "In collaboration with other agencies of the new administration, programs were mounted for malaria control in the South, rat control in the seaports, the sealing of abandoned mines to prevent stream pollution and . . . the construction of $5 million worth of rural privies."[8] Passage of the Social Security Act of 1935 was the most significant event in the reinvigoration of public health during the prewar period, providing for old-age benefits, public health services, and unemployment insurance. For the Public Health Service (PHS), the Social Security Act dramatically enhanced its capabilities, responsibilities, and mission. Titles V and VI of the act "provided millions for maternal and child health services and for public health in general. Social Security funds were channeled through the PHS, which in turn allocated them to the states based on their population and special needs. Social Security funding, along with other agencies' money for construction of health facilities and public works, dramatically raised the level of public health services throughout the

country."[1] As a consequence, the PHS assumed an important role in the recon-
struction of the United States after the Great Depression.

As a result of the New Deal, the PHS became embedded in the social fabric
of the nation in a more defined manner. During this period, the defining issues
for the PHS included such important tasks as making grants to states, cities,
and counties; battling over the issue of national health insurance; and measuring the health of various communities.[8] Federal funding became available for
the first time to train public health practitioners. The states were required to
publish minimum standards for public health practitioners, who were funded
through the new federal grant process. This process resulted in a move away
from the concept of employing any willing physician to conduct public health
activities and toward a system that required at least minimal public health
training. As a result, a number of universities developed schools or programs
of public health, and those that already existed expanded their programs significantly. The APHA's Committee on Professional Education determined that
in 1936, ten universities or schools of medicine in the United States and Canada provided at least one year of training to 346 individuals who received either a degree or a certificate of training in public health.[21] As a consequence,
the practice of public health was professionalized during the New Deal era.

Additional federal funding became available in the prewar years, directed
at specific diseases, programs, or populations. Thus, the categorical approach to
public health was born, a situation that continues to exist. "The categorical approach to public health proved politically popular. Members of Congress were
willing to allocate funds for specific diseases or for particular groups—health
and welfare services for children were especially favored—but they showed
less interest in general public health or administrative expenditures. Although
state health officers often felt constrained by targeted programs, they rarely re-
fused federal grants-in-aid and thus adapted their programs to the patterns of
available funds."[5] Throughout the decades to come, categorical funding would
become institutionalized and would shape the programs of public health departments across the country. Following the creation of the National Institutes
of Health, such categorical programs would shape its research agenda as well.

The onset of World War II resulted in the disruption of public health activities across the country as health departments lost personnel to the war effort, even though many were found unfit for military service due to a variety of
health-related issues. Special challenges were apparent as the increased number of men and women in uniform produced military camps and their distinctive issues, including a variety of infectious diseases. The PHS worked on
combating the prevalence of venereal diseases in the regions surrounding the
camps and addressed the prevalence of malaria in the South, particularly as it

impacted military training and operations. The Center for Controlling Malaria in the War Areas (forerunner to the Centers for Disease Control and Prevention [CDC]) was an effective tool in winning the battle against malaria in the southern United States. Other major victories over infectious diseases occurred during the war, particularly with the development of vaccines and the use of penicillin to treat wounded service members. The war's end brought a short-lived period of hope for an expanded public health agenda. Unfortunately, expansion of the PHS mission died aborning as the Cold War settled on the world at large, resulting in a dramatic change in American attitudes.

War on Poverty and Social Activism

In spite of numerous successes during the war years and afterward, as the 1950s drew to a close, it was obvious that a public health decline had reasserted itself. The funding of local health departments failed to keep pace with the increase in population.[22] By the end of the decade, federal grants to states had dropped by nearly 25 percent, from $45 million to $33 million. State and local health officers were inundated with a variety of new health issues, but due to funding and staff constraints, their responses were limited. As a result, their activities focused on the routine rather than the more important issues of the time. Woodcock noted, "Health departments are simply not doing the job. Without exception, state health and labor departments do not have the staff needed to enforce statutory standards of occupational health and safety."[23] In 1959 the APHA's Symposium on Politics and Public Health reported that "the full-time health officer is frequently, because of inadequate budget and staff, limited in his activities to a series of routine responsibilities. . . . In a great many areas the health officer position has been vacant year after year with little real hope of filling it. In these situations, even the pretense of public health leadership is left behind and local medical practitioners provide these clinical services on an hourly basis."[24] Mayor Raymond Tucker of St. Louis, the city hosting the APHA convention, stated that political opposition to public health programs often came from small but vocal politically powerful groups, and that although responsible public policy makers must consider public opinion, individuals must understand that such special-interest groups will always speak more loudly than those individuals supporting a program for the public good.[25] By the beginning of the 1960s, public health in the United States faced a dilemma. Once communicable infectious diseases had been controlled as a result of public health and medical interventions, a variety of noncommunicable diseases took their place among the leading causes of death—diseases with which the public health field was ill prepared to cope. At the same time, many public health officers failed to understand the importance of the political process.[26] The complacency of the 1950s gave way to the activism of the 1960s, including the War on Poverty and the civil rights movement. At the same time, the APHA underwent a metamorphosis as it expanded beyond its role as a professional organization serving its public health practitioner membership and began to engage in social action as an advocacy organization.

The War on Poverty, based on President Lyndon Johnson's Great Society, resulted in major new health programs, including the Medicare and Medicaid Acts of 1965. These new programs were designed to provide health care for individuals receiving Social Security benefits as well as for poor individuals and families. Significantly, these programs were directed at expanding individual medical care, leaving public health and its programs on the margin. "Most of the new health and social programs of the 1960s bypassed the structure of the public health agencies and set up new agencies to mediate between the federal government and local communities. Medicare and Medicaid reflected the usual priorities of the medical care system in favoring highly technical interventions and hospital care, while failing to provide adequately for preventive services."[5] Both programs, Medicare and Medicaid, bypassed the PHS.

The debate over Medicare focused on amending the Social Security Act instead of addressing the possibility that this new health care program might be developed under the auspices of public health. For more than a decade, the PHS had stood on the sidelines of the debates over national health care policy. Even PHS officials did not want to engage in what they believed would be simply an insurance scheme; thus, these key health care programs were lodged in other agencies of the Department of Health, Education, and Welfare.[8] Consequently, by the end of the 1960s, many of the broad functions of public health were dispersed among a variety of government agencies. "Losing a clear institutional base, public health had also lost visibility and clarity of definition."[5] The result for public health was disastrous and included a failure to engage public understanding and support for its mission.

Ferment of the 1970s and the Environmental Movement

The decade of the 1970s was filled with social upheaval that impacted public health and a variety of other American institutions. Throughout this decade, public health agencies slowly but surely became the clinical medical care providers of last resort for the uninsured, as well as for Medicaid recipients who were not accepted in the office practices of medical practitioners. Over the next decade and a half, health departments across the United States devoted nearly three-quarters of their funds from all sources to the direct clinical care of patients. The mission of public health, particularly prevention, suffered during this period as the provision of clinical care became all-encompassing. The public health infrastructure was starved of resources—staff, funds, and, above all, public support.[27] The 1970s also saw the rise of the environmental movement and other politically liberal endeavors. The Environmental Protection Agency was created, and the Clean Air Act of 1970 was enacted. Major public health agencies such as the Occupational Safety and Health Administration and the National Institute of Occupational Safety and Health were created, but as in the past, these agencies were located in other federal organizations. Clearly, public health agencies had failed to learn the importance of becoming politically adroit.

The Decline of Public Health

The decade of the 1980s was preceded by the Carter administration, which failed to establish a clear public health agenda. This four-year period was a forerunner to the Reagan administration, which tried to roll back the liberal agenda of the 1970s. The president's New Federalism resulted in many federal programs being "block-granted" back to state and local governments, with reduced budgets. These reductions could not have come at a more inopportune time, and the late 1970s to early 1980s constituted the nadir of modern public health in the United States. The one bright spot in the early 1980s was Reagan's nomination of C. Everett Koop as the fifteenth surgeon general of the U.S. Public Health Service. Following a difficult process that took nine months, Koop was confirmed by the Senate on November 16, 1981.[8] Arriving in Washington, D.C., Koop found the Public Health Service in deep disarray and realized that he would have "to reestablish the languishing authority of the Surgeon General and revive the morale of the Commissioned Corps."[28] While Koop was awaiting Senate confirmation, a new deadly public health menace arrived on the scene: AIDS. Initially, the Reagan administration tended to ignore the AIDS crisis, but Koop took the lead in informing the American public of the enormity of the threat. As the number of AIDS cases continued to rise, the PHS determined to send a letter from the surgeon general to every American household. At the time, "Understanding AIDS: A Message from the Surgeon General" held the record as "the largest print order and . . . the largest mailing in American history: 107,000,000 copies."[28] As a consequence, by the time he left office in 1989, Koop had completed his mission of revitalizing the PHS, and he had begun the process that would bring public health out of the "slough of despond" in which he had found it eight years before.

The impetus for raising public health from its 1980s nadir was the 1988 report of the Institute of Medicine (IOM) entitled *The Future of Public Health*. This seminal report laid the groundwork for public health's revitalization in the 1990s and beyond. It reflected a broad concern that public health's ebb was putting the nation's health in jeopardy. To quote the report, "This study was undertaken to address a growing perception among the Institute of Medicine membership and others concerned with the health of the public that this nation [has] lost sight of its public health goals and [has] allowed the system of public health activities to fall into disarray."[27] The report established that the public at large plays a significant role in maintaining an effective public health system. "In a free society, public activities ultimately rest on public understanding and support, not on the technical judgment of experts. Expertise is made effective only when it is combined with sufficient public support, a connection acted upon effectively by the early leaders of public health."[27] Since the role of public health had declined over the years, the IOM report summarized the current problems:

1. There is no clear, universally accepted mission for public health.
2. Tension between professional expertise and politics is present throughout the nation's public health system.
3. Public health professionals have been slow to develop strategies that demonstrate the worth of their efforts to legislators and the public.
4. Relationships between medicine and public health are uneasy, at best.
5. Inadequate research resources have been targeted at identifying and solving public health problems.
6. Public health practice, unlike other health professions, is largely decoupled from its academic bases.[29]

In addition, the report by the IOM's Committee for the Study of the Future of Public Health filled a need by setting out public health's previously undefined mission: "fulfilling society's interest in assuring conditions in which people can be healthy."[27] The committee defined the government's role in public health by establishing the core functions of public health agencies: assessment, policy development, and assurance.[27] The report began the process of rejuvenating public health in the United States.

A Period of Renaissance

Following the 1988 IOM report, the 1990s was a period of accelerated gains by public health. "In the late 1980s, many recognized that public health was limited in its ability to effectively deal with the onset of new and frightening problems, such as HIV/AIDS and multiple drug–resistant tuberculosis. These concerns led to a contemporary effort to better define public health responsibilities and bolster public health department capacity."[29] Following his inauguration in 1993, President Bill Clinton promised comprehensive health care reform. Although the president's initiative failed, his efforts to achieve health care reform, in combination with the IOM report, "acted as driving forces for the public health profession to better define its role and increase public understanding of its contributions to health."[28] These efforts resulted in a new sense of purpose and collaboration among a number of public health–related consortia, including governmental agencies at the federal, state, and local levels; various practitioner-related professional organizations; academic institutions; and individuals. Perhaps for the first time in its history, public health in the United States showed signs of becoming an academic discipline in its own right, even though schools of public health had been accredited as early as the mid-1940s. Initially, the core areas of public health had developed as separate academic disciplines, rather than public health as one overarching academic entity.

A major effort in this decade of consolidation was development of the list of ten essential public health services. In 1993 the CDC used the three core functions outlined in the IOM report—assessment, policy development, and assurance—to develop an expanded list of ten basic public health practices. This list was later refined by the Washington State Department of Health into a list of ten core functions. At the same time, a similar list was developed by the National Association of County Health Officials, the Association of State and Territorial Health Officials, and the U.S. Office of the Assistant Secretary for Health. In 1994 various organizations formed a working group to develop a consensus on the essential services of public health.[29] First, a short list was developed that described efforts to provide essential services to the public:

1. Prevent epidemics and the spread of disease.
2. Protect against environmental hazards.
3. Prevent injuries.
4. Promote and encourage healthy behaviors and mental health.
5. Respond to disasters and assist communities in recovery.
6. Assure the quality and accessibility of health services.[29]

A second list developed by the consensus group contained key descriptions of the ten essential public health services, and this has served as the guiding principle for the development of public health practices, services, and systems, as well as its academic framework:

1. Monitor health status to identify community health problems.
2. Diagnose and investigate health problems and health hazards in the community.
3. Inform, educate, and empower people about health issues.
4. Mobilize community partnerships to identify and solve health problems.
5. Develop policies and plans that support individual and community health efforts.
6. Enforce laws and regulations that protect health and ensure safety.
7. Link people to necessary personal health services and assure the provision of health care when it is otherwise unavailable.
8. Assure a competent public health and personal health care workforce.
9. Evaluate the effectiveness, accessibility, and quality of personal and population-based health services.
10. Research new insights and innovative solutions to health problems.[29]

The IOM report also galvanized the creation of the Faculty/Agency Forum, composed of a number of key organizations, including the APHA, Association of Schools of Public Health, Association of State and Territorial Health Officials, National Association of County Health Officials, and U.S. Conference of Local Health Officers. The forum was developed to consider the academic and educational component of the report, and by 1993, it had brought together the practice and academic communities to develop a list of competencies required for public health practice. "The Forum wanted to improve the quality of public health education and establish flourishing, permanent, broad cooperative agreements among schools of public health and major local, regional, and state public health agencies. To that end, the Forum also proposed ways that public agencies and institutions providing graduate education in public health could work together. After completing its work and publishing a report, the Forum went out of existence."[29] In follow-up efforts, the Council on Linkages was established in 1991, bringing together national public health organizations as well as the appropriate federal agencies to refine and implement the recommendations of its predecessor. The result of its work was the development of an up-to-date list of the core competencies required to practice public health as a discipline.[30-32] This effort led to a significant improvement in both academic public health education and in-service training.

The 1990s also saw the consolidation of the U.S. Conference of Local Health Officers and the National Association of County Health Officials into the National Association of County and City Health Officials (NACCHO), a professional organization involving the directors of all local health departments. This new organization focused greater attention on local health departments across the United States and their importance in developing public health policy. "In its new form, NACCHO is actively involved in developing public policy, its workforce, and leadership; defining and expanding the public health research agenda; developing tools to assist LHDs [local health departments] with community assessment; and providing technical assistance to public health practitioners."[29]

Another remarkable achievement in this period was the creation of the National Association of Local Boards of Health (NALBOH) in 1992. Earlier, local boards of health in some jurisdictions had developed associations to train new board members and help them address the issues of public health in their communities. NALBOH has grown rapidly and provides an appropriate venue for local support and training in such key areas as "legislative advocacy, emergency preparedness/terrorism, environmental health, oral health, the development of performance measurement standards, and tobacco control."[29]

Another organization added to the U.S. public health infrastructure was the Public Health Practice Program Office at the CDC, which, though formed in 1988, undertook its major efforts during this period of renaissance. It originally concentrated on four key public health areas: professional competencies, information systems, local health department organizational capacity, and development of the public health infrastructure science base. Later, a fifth area was added when the office developed science-based performance standards for public health organizations. Unfortunately, the office was disbanded in the late 1990s during a CDC reorganization.

The 1990s also saw renewed efforts to bring public health and medicine closer together. As far back as 1921 and their fight over the Sheppard-Towner Maternity and Infancy Protection Act, the fields of public health and medicine had been at odds. By 1996 the APHA and AMA teamed up to "bridge the gap and develop stronger working relationships between the two disciplines."[29] Several conferences were held, directed at developing collaborative practices. However, a number of shifting priorities intervened by the end of the decade and made continued collaboration difficult to sustain.

Toward the end of the 1990s, the Robert Wood Johnson Foundation and the W. K. Kellogg Foundation developed the Turning Point initiative in an effort "to transform the public health system in the United States to make the system more effective, more community-based, and more collaborative."[33] Although the initiative's funding ceased in 2006, its valuable contributions continue in a variety of formats. At the state level, Turning Point partners collaborated to influence good public health policy, expand information technology to make data available to local communities to address health concerns, and stimulate state agencies and organizations to develop comprehensive state health plans. Turning Point's National Excellence Collaborative worked to modernize public health statutes, create accountable systems to measure performance, utilize information technology, invest in social marketing, and develop leadership.[33]

An Awakened America

Public health, like all other aspects of American life, was jolted by the events of September 11, 2001. In the decade following the destruction of the World Trade Center in New York City and the attack on the Pentagon, public health was forever changed, yet it some ways, it continued unaltered. The new century's epidemic was terrorism and bioterrorism, and the response was public health preparedness. Slightly more than a year after the 9/11 attacks, the Department of Homeland Security was formed on November 25, 2002, and its primary responsibility is protecting the territory of the United States and responding to terrorist attacks, man-made accidents, and natural disasters (see http://www.dhs.gov). Soon after 9/11, the "mailing of letters contaminated with anthrax spores to certain media outlets and national governmental figures in the United States in early October 2001, [added] new urgency to terrorism preparedness activities."[29] As a result, state and local health departments worked tirelessly to develop the ability to respond to bioterrorism, which also improved their ability to respond to man-made and natural disasters. Former U.S. senator Sam Nunn noted that it was not until the 9/11 attacks that the issue of bioterrorism began to obtain the funding and attention it required. "In the event of a biological attack," he said, "millions of lives may depend on how quickly we diagnose the effects, report the findings, disseminate information to the healthcare communities and to state and local governments, and bring forth a fast and an effective response at the local, state, and federal levels. Public health must become an indispensable pillar of our national security framework."[34]

Over the next five years, the U.S. government appropriated approximately $5 billion "to introduce surveillance systems, purchase equipment, and develop plans, and, to some degree, measures" for public health preparedness.[35] The impact of Hurricane Katrina in 2005 galvanized national attention to the need for public health disaster preparedness, regardless of cause.[36] However, a major difficulty has been determining how to assess that preparedness. In 2007 Nelson and colleagues found that public health preparedness was not clearly defined and that without adequate means to assess performance, it was difficult to determine the effectiveness of federal funds expended. As a consequence, it was challenging "to assess the effectiveness of past investments, engage in continuous quality improvement of current efforts, or design and target future efforts."[37] A key factor in public health preparedness is crisis risk communication in public health emergencies. Since 9/11, public health practitioners have gained experience and skill in incorporating crisis risk communication into their practice of public health. However, public health communication is still a new and emerging field that requires the development of techniques to evaluate the effectiveness of crisis risk communication efforts.[38]

A major positive result of 9/11 has been the development of shared services among local public health systems. To illustrate, "regionalization in local public health has become increasingly common in the era of preparedness. Most states have responded to the challenge and funding for public health preparedness by setting up intrastate regional structures, but the rationale for these structures, the way they are implemented, and presumably their impact all vary widely."[39] Unfortunately, there is little evidence of interstate arrangements or larger regional public health emergency preparedness planning. Regionalization and mechanisms for shared police and fire services may be useful case studies for public health collaboration.[39] State and local public health agencies have developed working partnerships to improve surveillance and response capabilities at the state and local levels. However, as natural disasters such as Hurricane Katrina have demonstrated, broader regional and national emergency planning is required.

In his 2007 Shattuck lecture, Schroeder raised an important contemporary public health issue, stating that health disparities include unhealthy personal behaviors that are unevenly distributed in the U.S. population. As he cogently stated: "Improving population health would be more than a statistical accomplishment. It could enhance the productivity of the workforce and boost the national economy, reduce health care expenditures, and most important, improve people's lives."[40] In January 2000 the Department of Health and Human Services launched the *Healthy People 2010* initiative (a follow-up to *Healthy People 2000*), which committed the United States to the major goal of eliminating health disparities.[41, 42] "In recent decades, the improvement in health status has been remarkable for the U.S. population as a whole. However, racial and ethnic minority populations continue to lag behind whites with a quality of life diminished by illness from preventable chronic diseases and a life span cut short by premature death."[43] Socioeconomic disparities may be linked to health behaviors that are not conducive to good health. Tobacco use, physical inactivity, and poor nutrition produce health disparities that are not linked to the use of personal income to purchase good health.[44] At the same time, during the first decade of the twenty-first century, greater attention has been given to understanding these social determinants of health.[45] Engaging all the ramifications of health disparities, including the social determinants of the health of the population as a whole, has resulted in a clear public health agenda for the future.

To improve population health, public health relies almost entirely on government funding. Hemenway cites four reasons for the underfunding of public health: "First, the benefits of public health programs lie in the future. . . . Second, the beneficiaries of public health measures are generally unknown. . . . Third, in public health, the benefactors, too, are often unknown. . . . Fourth, some public health efforts encounter not just disinterest but out-and-out opposition."[46] Based on NACCHO data from 1997 and 2005, expenditures fell. "The total sum of local public health department expenditures per capita across all states was 15.8% lower in 2005 than 1997."[47] As a consequence, public health remained underfunded at the end of the first decade of the twenty-first century. Although there was new funding after the 9/11 attacks, "federal support for many other areas of public health programming diminished. Concomitant revenue shortfalls in many states actually led to reductions in funding for population-based public health services across the country. Instead of building capacity overall, public health agencies have been placed in the position of having to fund their basic services and the new preparedness expectations with what amounts to, in many cases, an overall reduction in funding."[29] Thus, a decade that began with high expectations that public health would become a key component of American life ended with mixed reviews. The key to the future of public health in America may well lie in the promotion of prevention, such as the 2010 Affordable Health Care Act enacted by Congress. "The Affordable Care Act creates a new Prevention and Public Health Fund to assist state and community efforts to prevent illness and promote health, so that all Americans can lead longer, more productive lives. The Fund represents an unprecedented investment—$15 billion over 10 years—that will help prevent disease, detect it early, and manage conditions before they become severe."[48] Koh and Sebelius believe that the act will revitalize prevention at all levels of society. It provides for four specific interventions: (1) providing "individuals with improved access to clinical preventive services," (2) promoting "wellness in the workplace and providing new health promotion opportunities for employers and employees," (3) strengthening "the vital role of communities in promoting prevention," and (4) elevating "prevention as a national priority and providing unprecedented opportunities for promoting health through all policies."[49] Thus, in the second decade of the twenty-first century, public health will continue to address some topics that have been pertinent for decades, and new ones will arise as the practice of public health continues to evolve in the United States.

Notes

1. Fee E, Brown TM. The unfilled promise of public health: Déjà vu all over again. *Health Aff.* 2002;21:31–43.

2. United States Congress. *An Act for the Relief of Sick and Disabled Seamen.* July 16, 1798 (I Stat. L., 605–606).

3. Powell JH. *Bring out Your Dead: The Great Plague of Yellow Fever in Philadelphia in 1793.* Philadelphia: University of Philadelphia Press; 1949.

4. Rosenberg CE. *The Cholera Years: The United States in 1832, 1849, and 1866.* Chicago: University of Chicago Press; 1962.

5. Fee E. History and development of public health. In: Scutchfield FD, Keck CW, eds. *Principles of Public Health Practice.* 3rd ed. Clifton Park, NY: Delmar; 2009.

6. Rosen G. *A History of Public Health.* Expanded edition. Baltimore: Johns Hopkins University Press; 1993.

7. Duffy J. *The Sanitarians: A History of American Public Health.* Urbana: University of Illinois Press; 1990.

8. Mullan F. *Plagues and Politics.* New York: Basic Books; 1989.

9. Markel H. *Quarantine! East European Jewish Immigrants and the New York City Epidemics of 1892.* Baltimore: Johns Hopkins University Press; 1997.

10. Rosenkrantz B. Cart before horse: Theory, practice, and professional image in American public health. *J Hist Med Allied Sci.* 1974;29:55–73.

11. Chapin C. How shall we spend the health appropriation? In: Chapin CV, Gorham FP, eds. *Papers of Charles V. Chapin, M.D.: A Review of Public Health Realities.* New York: Commonwealth Fund; 1934.

12. Williams RC. *The United States Public Health Service, 1798–1950.* Washington, DC: U.S. Government Printing Office; 1951.

13. Flexner A. *A Medical Education in the United States and Canada: A Report to the Carnegie Foundation for the Advancement of Teaching.* New York: Carnegie Foundation; 1910.

14. Welch WH, Rose W. Institute of Hygiene: Being a Report by Dr. William H. Welch and Wickliffe Rose to the General Education Board, Rockefeller Foundation; 1915. http://www.deltaomega.org/WelchRose.pdf. Accessed December 7, 2011.

15. Johnson P. *Modern Times: From the Twenties to the Nineties.* New York: HarperCollins; 1991.

16. Duffy J. The American medical profession and public health: From support to ambivalence. *Bull Hist Med.* 1979;53:1–22.

17. Winslow C-EA. Public health at the crossroads. *Am J Public Health.* 1999;89:1647.

18. Rosenkrantz B. *Public Health and the State: Changing Views in Massachusetts, 1842–1936.* Cambridge, MA: Harvard University Press; 1972.

19. Starr P. *The Social Transformation of American Medicine.* New York: Basic Books; 1982.

20. Committee on the Costs of Medical Care. *Medical Care for the American People: The Final Report of the Committee on the Costs of Medical Care.* Chicago: University of Chicago Press; 1932.

21. Leathers WS, et al. Public health degrees and certificates granted in 1936. *Am J Public Health.* 1937;27:1267–1272.

22. Sanders BS. Local health departments: Growth or illusion. *Public Health Rep.* 1959;74:13–20.

23. Woodcock L. Where are we going in public health? *Am J Public Health.* 1956;46:278–282.

24. Aronson JB. Reactions and summary: 1959 APHA symposium on politics and public health. *Am J Public Health.* 1959;49:311–313.

25. Tucker RR. The politics of public health. *Am J Public Health.* 1959;49:301–305.

26. Terris M. The changing face of public health. *Am J Public Health.* 1959;49:1113–1119.

27. Institute of Medicine, Committee for the Study of the Future of Public Health. *The Future of Public Health.* Washington, DC: National Academies Press; 1988.

28. Koop CE. *Koop: The Memoirs of America's Family Doctor.* Grand Rapids, MI: Zondervan; 1992.

29. Keck CW, Scutchfield FD. Emergence of a new public health. In: Scutchfield FD, Keck CW, eds. *Principles of Public Health Practice.* 3rd ed. Clifton Park, NY: Delmar; 2009.

30. Council on Linkages Public Health Research Project. http://www.phf.org/news/Pages/Core_Public_Health_Competencies_Use_Supported_by_Council_on_Linkages.aspx. Accessed July 21, 2011.

31. Association of Schools of Public Health. MPH Core Competency Model. Updated September 10, 2010. http://www.asph.org/document.cfm?page=851. Accessed July 21, 2011.

32. Association of Schools of Public Health. DrPH Core Competency Model. Released November 2009. http://www.asph.org/document.cfm?page=1004. Accessed July 21, 2011.

33. Turning Point. Collaborating for a New Century in Public Health. http://www.turningpointpartners.org. Accessed July 21, 2011.

34. Nunn S. The future of public health preparedness. *J Law Med Ethics.* 2002;30(3):202–209.

35. Seid M, Lotstein D, Williams VL, Nelson C, Leuschner KJ, Diamant A, Stern S, Wasserman J, Lurie N. Quality improvement in public health emergency preparedness. *Annu Rev Public Health.* 2002;28:19–31.

36. Lister SA. *Hurricane Katrina: The Public Health and Medical Response.* CRS Report for Congress. Washington, DC: Library of Congress, 2005.

37. Nelson C, Lurie N, Wasserman J. Assessing public health emergency preparedness: Concepts, tools, and challenges. *Annu Rev Public Health.* 2007;28:1–18.

38. Glik DC. Risk communication for public health emergencies. *Annu Rev Public Health.* 2007;28:33–54.

39. Koh HK, Elqura LJ, Judge CM, Stoto MA. Regionalization of local public health systems in the era of preparedness. *Annu Rev Public Health.* 2008;29:205–218.

40. Schroeder SA. We can do better—improving the health of the American people. *N Engl J Med.* 2007;357:1221–1228.

41. U.S. Department of Health and Human Services. *Healthy People 2010: Understanding and Improving Health.* 2nd ed. Washington, DC: DHHS; 2000.

42. Carter-Pokras O, Baquet C. What is a "health disparity"? *Public Health Rep.* 2001;117:426–434.

43. Thomas SB, Quinn SC, Butler J, Fryer CS, Garza A. Toward a fourth generation of disparities research to achieve health equity. *Annu Rev Public Health.* 2011;32:399–416.

44. Pampel FC, Krueger PM, Denney JT. Socioeconomic disparities in health behaviors. *Annu Rev Public Health.* 2010;36:349–370.

45. Braveman P, Egerter S, Williams DR. The social determinants of health: Coming of age. *Annu Rev Public Health.* 2011;32:381–398.

46. Hemenway D. Why we don't spend enough on public health. *N Engl J Med.* 2010;362:1657–1658.

47. Arnett PK. *Local Health Department Changes over the Past Twenty Years.* Unpublished dissertation; 2011.

48. Healthcare.gov. The Affordable Care Act's Prevention and Public Health Fund in Your State. Posted February 9, 2011. http://www.healthcare.gov/news/factsheets/prevention020920111a.html. Accessed August 11, 2011.

49. Koh HK, Sebelius KG. Promoting prevention through the affordable care act. *N Engl J Med.* 2011;363:1296–1299.

1

The Social and Ecological Determinants of Health

Steven H. Woolf and Paula Braveman

In 2003 the landmark report *Unequal Treatment* drew the nation's attention to disparities in the way health care is delivered to racial or ethnic minority groups.[1] Studies had documented that patients with similar clinical presentations but different races or ethnicities received different clinical recommendations and different levels of clinical care. The report also documented disparities in access to care and health insurance coverage. The health care system responded by launching a variety of initiatives to study the issue, standardize care delivery, heighten providers' cultural competency, and increase minority representation among health care professionals. The effort to expand access to medical care and health insurance coverage has been a central theme of health care reform.

Although these efforts have yielded some progress in reducing disparities in health care,[2] disparities in health itself persist. African American infants are twice as likely as white infants to die before their first birthday, a ratio that has been nearly the same for more than forty years.[3, 4] Between 1960 and 2000 the standardized mortality ratio for blacks relative to whites changed little, from 1.472 in 1960 to 1.412 in 2000, and by 2002 there were an estimated 83,750 excess deaths in the United States among blacks.[4] The maternal mortality rate is also higher among some racial and ethnic minority groups.[5] For example, black women were around 3.4 times as likely as white women to die of pregnancy-related causes in 2006—a difference of 32.7 versus 9.5 maternal deaths for every 100,000 live births.[6]

In the "Eight Americas" study, Murray and colleagues divided the U.S. population into eight groups: Asians (America 1), below-median-income whites living in the Northland (America 2), Middle Americans (America 3),

Table 1.1. Life Expectancy of Eight Demographic Subgroups in the United States

America	General Description	Male Life Expectancy at Birth (yrs)	Female Life Expectancy at Birth (yrs)	Female–Male Difference in Life Expectancy (yrs)
1	Asian	82.8	87.7	4.9
2	White low-income rural Northland	76.2	81.8	5.6
3	Middle America	75.2	80.2	5.0
4	White poor Appalachia/ Mississippi Valley	71.8	77.8	6.0
5	Western Native American	69.4	75.9	6.5
6	Black Middle America	69.6	75.9	6.3
7	Black poor rural South	67.7	74.6	6.9
8	Black high-risk urban	66.7	74.9	8.2

Source: Murray CJ, Kulkarni S, Ezzati M. Eight Americas: New perspectives on U.S. health disparities. *Am J Prev Med.* 2005;29(5 Suppl 1):4–10.

poor whites living in Appalachia and the Mississippi Valley (America 4), Native Americans living on reservations in the West (America 5), black Middle Americans (America 6), poor blacks living in the rural South (America 7), and blacks living in high-risk urban environments (America 8).[7] For males, the difference in life expectancy between America 1 and America 8 was 16.1 years (table 1.1), as large as the gap between Iceland, which had the highest male life expectancy in the world, and Bangladesh.[7]

Health disparities are just as large in some cities of the United States. For example, in Orleans Parish (New Orleans), life expectancy varies by 25.5 years between zip codes. In zip code 70112—the neighborhoods of Tulane, Gravier, Iberville, Treme, and the central business district of New Orleans—life expectancy is 54.5 years,[8] comparable to the 2009 life expectancy reported by Congo (55 years), Nigeria (54 years), and Uganda (52 years).[9]

Health disparities related to race and ethnicity persist even among patients in health care systems that offer similar levels of access to care and coverage benefits, such as the Veterans Health Administration and Kaiser Permanente integrated health care systems.[10, 11] This evidence tells us that the causes of and solutions to such disparities lie beyond health care.

Determinants of Health and Health Disparities

Understanding the causes of health disparities requires an understanding of the determinants of health itself. Morbidity and mortality are influenced by intrinsic biological factors such as age, sex, and genetic characteristics. Some other risk factors that affect health are referred to as "downstream" determinants because they are often shaped by "upstream" societal conditions. For example, medical care is important, particularly when people become ill, but other factors influence whether people become ill and their resilience and response to treatment. Personal behaviors and actions—such as tobacco use, seeking medical care for chest pain or other health complaints, and adherence to providers' recommendations—also affect health outcomes. Fully 38 percent of all deaths in the United States have been attributed to four health behaviors: tobacco use, diet, physical activity, and problem drinking.[12] Some health problems are produced directly through environmental exposures to physical risks, such as respiratory illness induced by air and water pollution, foodborne infections, injuries sustained in motor vehicle crashes, and the physical and mental trauma resulting from crime.[13, 14]

However, exposure to these immediate, or proximate, health risks is itself shaped by the context or conditions in which people live—the distal or "upstream" determinants of health.[15-22] Living conditions influence the degree to which people are exposed to environmental risks, can pursue healthy behaviors, or are able to obtain quality medical care.[23-26] What are known as *social determinants of health*—personal resources such as education and income and the social environment in which people live, work, study, and play—influence whether people become ill and the severity of illness.[27] They affect access to health care but also patients' vulnerability to illness and their ability to care for conditions at home. Social determinants provide an important key to understanding health disparities in the United States and, as this chapter explains, are themselves the product of more upstream societal influences.

The Interaction of Education and Income

The relationship between affluence and health has been described throughout history. In modern times, the Whitehall studies from the 1970s in the United Kingdom and decades of subsequent research throughout the world have documented large health inequities associated with social class and occupation.[28] The most familiar social determinants in the United States are income and education. Adults living in poverty are more than five times as likely to report only fair or poor health compared with adults whose incomes are at least four times the poverty level.[29] In adults, serious psychological distress is more than five times as common among the poor.[3] Men and women in the highest income group can expect to live at least 6.5 years longer than poor men and women.[20]

The relationship between income and health is not restricted to the poor.

Table 1.2. Self-Reported Health by Income, Race, and Ethnicity

Race/Ethnicity	<100% FPL*	100–199% FPL	200–299% FPL	300–399% FPL	≥ 400% FPL
Black, non-Hispanic	36.1	26.3	18.0	14.4	9.8
Hispanic	29.6	22.5	16.7	13.2	9.7
White, non-Hispanic	30.8	20.7	13.5	9.5	6.2

Note: Values refer to the proportion of adults aged 25 years and older who described their health as "fair" or "poor."
Source: Braveman P, Egerter S. *Overcoming Obstacles to Health.* Princeton, NJ: Robert Wood Johnson Foundation; 2008.
*FPL, federal poverty level.

Studies of Americans at all income levels reveal inferior health status in lower versus higher income strata (table 1.2).[20] For example, the life expectancy of a 25-year-old with a family income that is 400 percent or more of the poverty level (more than $87,000 per year for a family of four in 2009) is 55.7 years, with progressively shorter life expectancies as family income declines: 53.8 years with an income 200 to 399 percent of the poverty level, 51.4 years with an income 100 to 199 percent of the poverty level, and 49.2 years with an income less than 100 percent of the poverty level. The same health gradient by income is apparent in the prevalence rates for coronary heart disease, diabetes, and activity limitations due to chronic disease. Even those with incomes at 300 to 399 percent of the poverty level have worse health outcomes than those with incomes of 400 percent or greater.[20]

This pattern is of great importance to the large and growing middle-class population of the United States. A common misconception among the public and policy makers is that health outcomes are compromised only for those few members of the population living at the extremes of social disadvantage. The mistaken belief is that only those living in extreme poverty or in oppressed urban neighborhoods, in rural areas, or on Native American reservations are confronted by living conditions of sufficient severity to affect health. Yet the scientific evidence documents a clear income gradient and dose-response relationship between income or wealth and health, suggesting that all members of the population, including the middle class, experience inferior health outcomes compared with more affluent members. Current economic trends are expanding the size of the middle class in the United States (see later), and the adverse health risks they experience carry increased public health implications.

That income is important to health may not be surprising to some, but the magnitude of the relationship is not always recognized. For example, Krieger and colleagues reported that 14 percent of premature deaths among whites and 30 percent of premature deaths among blacks between 1960 and 2002 would not have occurred if all persons had experienced the mortality rates of whites in the highest income quintile.[30] Woolf and associates reported that 25 percent of all deaths in Virginia between 1996 and 2002 would have been averted if the mortality rates of the five most affluent counties and cities existed statewide.[31] Muennig and colleagues estimated that living at less than 200 percent of the federal poverty level claimed more than 400 million quality-adjusted life years between 1997 and 2002, a larger effect than tobacco use and obesity.[32] These estimates all rely on assumptions about causality that ignore the influence of confounding variables, but they suggest that the confluence of conditions existing among people with limited income exerts a much greater health influence than is widely appreciated.

An important pathway to income is education, and the literature documents profound health disparities among adults with different levels of educational attainment. Adults who lack a high school education or equivalent are three times more likely to die before age 65 than those with a college education.[33] The average 25-year-old male with less than 12 years of education can expect to live almost 7 fewer years than someone with at least 16 years of education.[20] Infants born to mothers with greater education are less likely to die before their first birthday. For the years 1988–2007, the infant mortality rate was 4.2 per 1,000 live births for mothers who graduated from college, but 7.8 per 1,000 live births for those who did not graduate from high school.[33] Such parents are approximately four times more likely to describe their children's health as good, fair, or poor than are parents who are college graduates.[20, 33]

According to Elo and Preston's multivariate analysis of National Longitudinal Mortality Survey data, every additional year of educational attainment reduces the odds of dying at age 35 to 54 years by 1 to 3 percent.[34] Jemal and colleagues calculated that 48 percent of all male deaths and 38 percent of all female deaths in 2001 occurring in those aged 25 to 64 years would not have occurred if the population had experienced the death rates of college graduates.[35] Woolf and associates estimated that giving all U.S. adults the mortality rate of adults with some college education would have saved seven lives for every life saved by biomedical advances between 1996 and 2002.[36]

Reflecting the historical legacy of discrimination, evidence documents stark racial and ethnic differences in education and income that could—given the health benefits associated with educational attainment—explain the inferior health status experienced by blacks and other minority groups. In 2008 the high school dropout rate among 16- to 24-year-olds was 18.3 percent for Hispanics, almost four times the rate for non-Hispanic whites (4.8 percent) and almost twice the rate for blacks (9.9 percent). In 2009 the proportion of Hispanic adults (aged 25 and older) with less than 7 years of elementary school education (kindergarten to eighth grade) was 16.5 percent, twenty times the rate for non-Hispanic whites (0.8 percent). By 2010 the percentage of adults aged 25 and older who had obtained a bachelor's degree or higher education had reached 33.2 percent among whites but was only 20.0 percent among blacks and 13.9 percent among Hispanics.[33]

Americans' income and wealth also differ markedly by race and ethnicity. In 2009 the median household income of blacks and Hispanics—$32,584 and $38,039, respectively—was roughly two-thirds the income of non-Hispanic whites ($54,461).[37] Net worth—the sum of assets minus debts—also differed markedly by race and ethnicity. A report by the Pew Charitable Trust, based on an analysis of 2009 data collected by the U.S. Census Bureau, documented that white households had twenty times the net worth of black households and eighteen times the net worth of Hispanic households.[38] In 2009 the poverty rate among blacks and Hispanics was 25.8 and 25.3 percent, respectively, almost three times the rate among non-Hispanic whites (9.4 percent).[37]

Education and income are related to health in complex ways, partly because they are interrelated (e.g., people with more education generally have higher earnings).[39] Education and income are elements of a complex web of interwoven social and economic conditions that exert health effects over a lifetime.[40] These conditions include employment, wealth, neighborhood characteristics, and social policies, as well as culture, health beliefs, and country of origin. A variety of models have been proposed to illustrate the layers of influences that interact in shaping health outcomes.[41] The socioecological model is one such framework, as is an elegant conceptual model developed by the Robert Wood Johnson Foundation's Commission to Build a Healthier America.[42] Figure 1.1 presents the conceptual framework adopted by the World Health Organization's Commission on Social Determinants of Health.[18]

Because of the complex interrelationships among the various social determinants of health, caution is required when drawing inferences about observed associations between health outcomes and isolated variables such as education or income. Such associations are subject to confounding by related factors and require more sophisticated analyses that adjust for multivariate influences and interaction effects. Researchers are using longitudinal studies and advanced analytic techniques such as multilevel and structural equation modeling to help disentangle confounding variables and quantify the individual contributions of different factors to health outcomes. Even with such

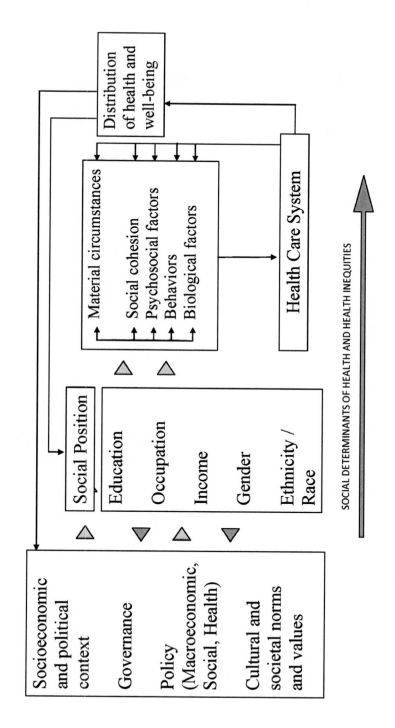

Figure 1.1. Conceptual framework of WHO Commission on Social Determinants of Health. *Source:* Commission on Social Determinants of Health. *Closing the Gap in a Generation: Health Equity through Action on the Social Determinants of Health.* Final Report of the Commission on Social Determinants of Health. Geneva: World Health Organization; 2008.

adjustments, the cumulative body of evidence affirms the important role of education and income as leading health predictors.

What could explain these associations? Lack of education increases one's likelihood of unemployment or low income, and both are associated with lack of health insurance and inability to pay for medical expenses. People with limited education and income may also be more likely to engage in unhealthy behaviors. As of 2009, the prevalence of smoking was 28.9 percent among adults without a high school diploma or equivalent, more than triple the rate among college graduates (9.0 percent).[3] Explanations for such associations vary. A good education might offer students skills and knowledge that help discourage smoking. For example, people with low literacy might not fully absorb messages about the harms of smoking, or they might be unable to afford or lack insurance coverage for cessation services or pharmacologic aids. To some extent, however, education and income are also linked to unhealthy behaviors through more complicated causal pathways. Research suggests that socioeconomic inequalities in health are only partly explained by health behaviors.[43-45] For example, the social and physical environments of people with low socioeconomic status may promote unhealthy behaviors in part because they are stressful.[46-48]

The Role of Neighborhoods and Communities

Unhealthy behaviors are partly matters of personal choice, but extensive evidence documents that they are also strongly influenced by the environment.[20, 22, 23, 27, 49] One might desire a healthy diet but be unable to afford nutritious foods or live too far from a supermarket that sells fresh fruits and vegetables.[22, 50-54] Parents might want to limit their children's screen time and encourage outdoor physical activity, but their neighborhoods may lack green space or sidewalks, or crime may be a concern. Walking to the store or cycling to work is unrealistic if the *built environment*—the design of roads, overpasses, and pedestrian routes—discourages physical activity. Poor and minority neighborhoods are often "food deserts" with limited access to healthy foods and a dense concentration of fast-food outlets and corner stores and bodegas that market inexpensive, calorie-rich foods.[55, 56] Liquor stores and conspicuous advertising for tobacco and alcohol are more common in depressed neighborhoods than in advantaged areas.[57] Schools in neighborhoods that produce little property tax revenue[58] often serve cafeteria meals consisting of less expensive high-calorie foods, or they may generate funds from vending machines stocked with soft drinks and candy.[59] In these settings, social norms may reinforce unhealthy behaviors. In short, healthy behaviors partly reflect personal choice, but they also require supportive resources and environments.[60]

But behaviors are not the whole story.[61-63] Distressed neighborhoods can induce disease and foment health disparities via pathways unrelated to personal health behaviors.[64-66] For example, a neighborhood's housing can be unhealthy, exposing occupants to lead, asbestos, and allergens that cause or worsen asthma and other respiratory illnesses. Bus depots, factories, highways, and hazardous waste sites are often situated near low-income neighborhoods or communities of color.[67, 68]

Social conditions are also important. Health may be compromised by the chronic stress of living amid a multitude of adverse environmental conditions, such as concentrated poverty, unemployment, urban blight, and crime.[21] Residents in such settings may be less able to connect with and support their neighbors; inadequate social cohesion is thought to have an independent adverse effect on health.[69, 70]

Highly segregated minority communities often face multiple obstacles to healthy living. For example, communities of color are the targets of captivating advertising, often directed at minority youth, to promote alcohol and tobacco products and the sale of high-calorie foods and beverages.[41, 71-74] In these highly segregated neighborhoods, this occurs against a larger backdrop in which the vestiges of racism and social exclusion may have their own health implications.[75-79] Victims of perceived discrimination—past and present—face a complex tableau of sociological consequences that may affect health, ranging from lack of trust in health care providers to psychic injury as victims of long-standing prejudice.[80]

Entrenched patterns reflecting long-standing disadvantage in low-income and minority neighborhoods often perpetuate cycles of socioeconomic failure.[81-83] Depressed neighborhoods often lack employment opportunities. There may be a shortage of health care providers, giving residents limited access to primary, specialty, and ancillary medical services. Low-income residents often cannot afford to move to a better neighborhood. Even commuting across town to find a (better) job, a supermarket, or a good doctor may be difficult if public transportation is unavailable or too costly.

Biological Pathways to Health Disparities

Galea and colleagues recently estimated that 245,000 of all deaths in 2000 were attributable to low education, 176,000 to racial segregation, 162,000 to low social support, 133,000 to individual-level poverty, and 119,000 to income inequality.[84] How do these conditions claim lives? Research has identified several plausible biological pathways. For example, stress—especially the chronic stress experienced by people confronting the challenges of living with inadequate resources on a daily basis—can produce neuroendocrine effects, such as the production of higher levels of cortisol and epinephrine, which can alter immune function and cause inflammation, among other outcomes. Although acute exposure to these substances may be harmless, repeated or sustained exposure over time is thought to produce "wear and tear" on organ systems and may precipitate chronic diseases such as diabetes and cardiovascular disease.[85]

The most impactful health effects of social and behavioral conditions may not be immediate. A growing body of evidence indicates that such effects unfold over a lifetime.[86] Experiences in utero and in early childhood, including stress, can have lasting effects that do not manifest until late adulthood—or perhaps not even until the next generation. An adult mother's childhood experiences can leave a biological imprint that affects the health and the neurological and mental development of her offspring. Infant health is no longer seen as the product of prenatal care alone, which actually has only a weak correlation with birth outcomes;[87] nor can adult health be viewed solely as the product of adult experiences.[86] Even the effects of genes are subject to environmental influences. Advances in the discipline known as epigenetics have shown that the social and physical environment can determine whether a gene for a disease is expressed (activated) or remains silent.[21] A person's epigenetic makeup may be transmitted to offspring. Increasingly, the biologically plausible pathways that link social determinants to health outcomes are becoming clear.

Declining Income and Increasing Inequality

Given that income plays a major role in health disparities, it is worrisome that income in the United States has been declining since 1999. Between 1999 and 2009 median household income in the United States decreased from $52,388 to $49,777. Other signs of economic hardship are apparent. The poverty rate has increased from 11.3 percent in 2000 to 14.3 percent in 2009—the highest rate since 1994 and the largest absolute number on record.[37] Between 2000 and 2009 the number of households with food insecurity increased from 10 million to 17 million. The proportion of people with severe housing cost burdens (spending more than 50 percent of their income on housing) increased from 13 percent in 2001 to more than 18 percent in 2009. The number of homeless families increased from 474,000 in 2007 to 535,000 in 2009.[37]

Some research suggests that health disparities are generated not only by low absolute levels of income but also by the degree of economic inequality in a society—the gap between rich and poor.[21, 88] Although this hypothesis remains unproved in the scientific literature, Richard Wilkinson and other investigators have written extensively on the topic and have demonstrated with the use of several indices that nations with higher levels of income inequality appear to have worse health outcomes and other measures of well-being.[89] However, other scientists have questioned whether such associations take full account of confounding variables such as absolute income levels and other measures of material deprivation. Whether income inequality alone, separate from other highly related variables, is an independent cause of shorter life expectancy and inferior health outcomes is not entirely certain.

There is, however, little debate that income inequality is increasing in the industrialized world, especially in the United States. The gap between the rich and the poor has been widening for decades. The Gini coefficient, a common measure of income inequality, has been increasing since 1968. The ratio between household income at the 90th and 10th percentiles increased steadily between 1999 and 2009. Only a small subset of affluent Americans saw their earnings grow over time; the remainder experienced a decline, a trend that accelerated after the economic turmoil produced by the 2007 recession.[36, 37]

The adverse impact of the recession on the net worth of Americans was documented in a 2011 report by the Pew Charitable Trust, which examined data from the U.S. Census Bureau's Survey of Income and Program Participation. It found that between 2005 and 2009, the share of wealth held by the top 10 percent increased from 49 to 56 percent. Over the same years, the inflation-adjusted median net worth for all white households fell by 16 percent, from $134,992 to $113,149. Minorities experienced even greater declines in net worth, which fell by 66 percent among Hispanic households (from $18,359 to $6,325) and 53 percent among black households (from $12,124 to $5,677).[38]

That the average American is losing income and wealth carries important health implications. In 1980 the United States ranked fourteenth in life expectancy relative to other industrialized countries, but since then, the U.S. ranking has progressively declined. By 2008 the United States ranked twenty-fifth in life expectancy, behind Portugal and Slovenia.[90] Likewise, infant mortality rates and other health indicators have not kept pace with those of other industrialized countries. The infant mortality rate in the United States is not only higher than that of most affluent nations but also higher than that of Cuba, a country with far lower per capita economic resources.[91]

The downturn in health status in the United States relative to other industrialized nations has several possible explanations. For example, a National Research Council study that compared international data for adults aged 50 and older concluded that an important reason for the U.S. failure to keep pace with other nations' life expectancy gains was that, in the past generation, cigarette smoking rates were higher in the United States than in other countries.[92] Other proposed explanations include the higher prevalence of obesity in the United States and deficiencies in the U.S. health care system in terms of quality, equity, and patient satisfaction. A particular concern among health services researchers is that Americans tend to have less access to primary care services than do citizens of other industrialized nations, a factor that is thought to have important health implications.[93]

However, a persistent question is whether health status in the United States is slipping because of unfavorable societal and economic conditions. Other industrialized countries outperform the United States in terms of educating students, and they have lower child poverty rates. For example, the United Nations Children's Fund (UNICEF) reports that the percentage of children (aged 0 to 17 years) living in families with incomes less than 50 percent of the nation's median income is higher in the United States than in any of the twenty-three other industrialized nations in the Organization for Economic Cooperation and Development (OECD) (figure 1.2).[94] Other countries also appear to have stronger safety nets, providing resources to help poor and

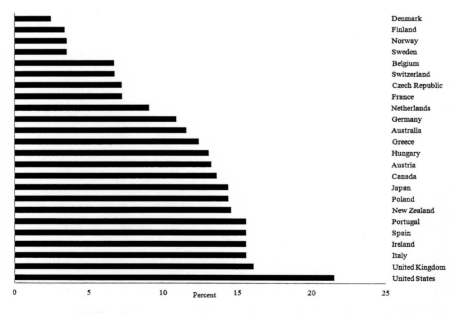

Figure 1.2. Childhood poverty rates in twenty-four member countries of the Organization for Economic Cooperation and Development. *Source:* UNICEF. *Child Poverty in Perspective: An Overview of Child Well-Being in Rich Countries.* Innocenti Research Centre Report Card 7. Florence: United Nations Children's Fund; 2007.

disadvantaged families maintain their health and cope with adversity. Other societies contribute a larger tax base to programs that provide aid to the unemployed, maternal and children's services, welfare assistance, and education and job training. Employment benefits appear to be more favorable for workers in other countries.[95, 96]

The Upstream Role of Policies, Macroeconomics, and Societal Structure

The social safety net, the conditions of neighborhoods, and access to education and income are parameters set by society, not by physicians, hospitals, health plans, or even the public health community. The agents of change who can make the most substantial improvements in public health may be the decision makers outside of health care who are positioned to strengthen schools, enhance child care, promote college education, reduce unemployment, improve job markets, teach workers marketable skills, stabilize the economy, and restore neighborhood infrastructure. Health disparities tied to income and wealth can be softened by health care leaders—for example, expanding health insurance coverage and lowering co-payments are important—but the more fundamental solution is for people to obtain better jobs and higher earnings, investments, and savings. Efforts are needed to reduce food insecurity and precarious housing, ensure universal access to quality education from preschool through college, support families with young children, and invest in affordable housing and transportation.

Even the public health endeavors to encourage smoking cessation and reduce obesity teach that policy often achieves more than clinical intervention. Progress in reducing tobacco use in the past 20 years has been less about counseling smokers to quit than about implementing public policies to restrict indoor smoking and increase cigarette prices.[97–101] The most influential change agents to promote healthy diets and physical activity may be the agencies and business interests that determine advertising messages, supermarket locations, school lunch menus, the content of food supplements provided through public programs such as after-school and summer sports programs, food labeling for fat and caloric content, and the built environment.[102] Key participants include city planners, state officials, federal agencies, legislatures, employers, school boards, zoning commissions, developers, supermarket chains, restaurants, and industries that range from beverage manufacturers to transit companies. Initiatives by hospitals, medical societies, and insurers to reduce health care disparities remain vital, but the front line in narrowing health disparities may lie beyond health care.

The "Health-in-All-Policies" Movement

Communities are learning from experience that "nonhealth" policies—those that once seemed unrelated to medicine or public health, such as transportation, housing, education, labor, tax, and land use policies—are important to maintaining population health and reducing health disparities. The "health-in-all-policies" movement encourages policy makers to consider how the health of the general public and vulnerable populations might be affected by proposed policies, regulations, or legislation. This approach helps address health disparities, such as when urban planners demolish an abandoned warehouse complex and use the land for a public park or the city council enacts zoning provisions or tax incentives to persuade a supermarket to locate in a "food desert" neighborhood. Health impact assessments—analyses that estimate the potential health benefits and harms associated with proposed policies—are now being commissioned to examine the health consequences of policies ranging from minimum-wage laws to freeway expansion and utility permits.[103–105]

The health-in-all-policies approach has been adopted by large and small communities throughout the United States and at the state level. The governor of California established the Health in All Policies Task Force in 2010.[106] At the federal level, the health-in-all-policies approach is evident in initiatives by the Obama administration and in provisions of the Affordable Care Act that promote interagency collaboration and coordination on cross-sector policies related to healthy housing, obesity, and other public health priorities.[107]

This new policy direction comes at the recommendation of blue-ribbon commissions sponsored by the World Health Organization,[18] the MacArthur Foundation,[19] the Robert Wood Johnson Foundation,[108] and the Institute of Medicine[109]—all of which have emphasized the importance of social determinants of health. Studies in the Bay Area of California, New York City, and other locales have used geospatial mapping techniques to document striking health disparities between census tracts and their strong and ubiquitous association with local social and environmental conditions. The notion that "place matters" to health was eloquently evoked by the acclaimed 2008 documentary film *Unnatural Causes*,[110] and that idea has become the organizing focus of initiatives by the W. K. Kellogg Foundation, the California Endowment, and the Robert Wood Johnson Foundation to press for changes at the local level to address health-related living conditions.

The fundamental role of these conditions as root causes of health disparities underscores the fallacy of viewing disparities as primarily the product of voluntary personal choices or of a health care system that treats patients unfairly.

Initiatives by hospitals, medical societies, and insurers remain vital, but an emerging focus in medicine and public health must be on education, vibrant communities, and other social conditions as key elements of a strategy to achieve health equity. Needed reforms to health care delivery should not mask the reality that the root causes of disparities in health (and in health care) lie outside the walls of hospitals, ambulatory care practices, and nursing homes.

Nor should resources for rectifying disparities, either through policy and service programs or through scientific research, be concentrated on health care to the exclusion of understanding and improving the upstream conditions responsible for disparities. Befitting the importance of the issue, the National Institutes of Health and other funders have issued a larger number of grants to study the social determinants of health, but the vast majority of research on racial and ethnic disparities continues to be concentrated on care delivery, health insurance coverage, minority representation in the clinical workforce, and access to care providers.

A challenge to research funders with traditional interests in conventional topics in medicine and public health is that social determinants do not fit comfortably within the nominal boundaries of the health sector, let alone the organ systems or disease categories that shape the focus and funding of most health research. Studies conducted by schools of education, business, urban design, or social work, as well as research on interventions to improve employment, wages, housing, or land use, are peripheral to the interests of most of the federal health agencies and nonprofit foundations that fund the vast majority of public health or health services research. Entities that fund research in the social sciences, economics, and business may not be accustomed to receiving applications from medical schools or public health researchers, and they may be unfamiliar with the analytic methods or terminology used by biomedical investigators.

There are equally problematic challenges in the policy sector, where social determinants of health lack a natural home. For example, legislatures and executive branch agencies in the federal and state governments are accustomed to delegating health issues to committees that deal with medicine, public health, Medicare, or Medicaid. Nonhealth issues such as college scholarships, jobless rates, and municipal development fall under the auspices of committees and agencies that deal with labor, taxes, commerce, agriculture, transportation, and so on. Typically, neither the members nor the staffs of health committees or agencies are equipped to take up education reform, transportation policy, job growth, and other nonhealth policies as strategies to improve health or reduce health disparities. More typically, public discourse about *health* often succumbs to the strong gravitational pull of *health care:* the public and policy makers look to health care to solve health problems, as do many members of the health care community.

An ongoing challenge for the public health community will be to reinforce the message that health is determined by more than health care and to articulate the argument for connecting social and economic policies to health outcomes and medical spending. The health argument alone is unlikely to succeed in overcoming the daunting political obstacles, but it may make an important contribution when added to other arguments based on both economic concerns and a commitment to social justice.

Notes

1. Smedley BD, Stith AY, Nelson AR, eds. *Unequal Treatment: Confronting Racial and Ethnic Disparities in Health Care.* Committee on Understanding and Eliminating Racial and Ethnic Disparities in Health Care, Board on Health Sciences Policy, Institute of Medicine. Washington, DC: National Academies Press; 2003.

2. Agency for Healthcare Research and Quality. *2010 National Healthcare Disparities Report.* AHRQ Publication No. 11-0005. Rockville, MD: U.S. Department of Health and Human Services; 2011.

3. National Center for Health Statistics. *Health, United States, 2010: With Special Feature on Death and Dying.* Hyattsville, MD; 2011.

4. Satcher D, Fryer GE Jr, McCann J, Troutman A, Woolf SH, Rust G. What if we were equal? A comparison of the black-white mortality gap in 1960 and 2000. *Health Aff.* 2005;24(2):459–464.

5. Chang J, Elam-Evans LD, Berg CJ, Herndon J, Flowers L, Seed KA, Syverson CJ. Pregnancy-related mortality surveillance—United States, 1991–1999. *MMWR Surveill Summ.* 2003;52(2):1–8.

6. Heron M, Hoyert DL, Murphy SL, et al. Deaths: Final data for 2006. *National Vital Statistics Reports.* April 17, 2009;57(14):2, 13. www.cdc.gov/nchs/data/nvsr57/nvsr57_14.pdf.

7. Murray CJ, Kulkarni S, Ezzati M. Eight Americas: New perspectives on U.S. health disparities. *Am J Prev Med.* 2005;29(5 Suppl 1):4–10.

8. *Social Determinants of Health and Crime in Post-Katrina Orleans Parish.* Richmond: Virginia Commonwealth University Center on Human Needs; 2011.

9. World Health Organization. World health statistics. http://www.who.int/whosis/whostat/EN_WHS2011_Part2.xls. Accessed September 6, 2011.

10. Saha S, Freeman M, Toure J, Tippens KM, Weeks C, Ibrahim S. Racial and ethnic disparities in the VA health care system: A systematic review. *J Gen Intern Med.* 2008;23:654–671.

11. Sandel ME, Wang H, Terdiman J, Hoffman JM, Ciol MA, Sidney S, Quesenberry C, Lu Q, Chan L. Disparities in stroke rehabilitation: Results of a study in an integrated health system in northern California. *PMR.* 2009;1:29–40.

12. Mokdad AH, Marks JS, Stroup DF, Gerberding JL. Actual causes of death in the United States, 2000. *JAMA.* 2004;291:1238–1245.

13. Morello-Frosch R, Zuk M, Jerrett M, Shamasunder B, Kyle AD. Understanding the cumulative impacts of inequalities in environmental health: Implications for policy. *Health Aff.* 2011;30:879–887.

14. Jakubowski B, Frumkin H. Environmental metrics for community health improvement. *Prev Chronic Dis.* 2010;7(4):A76.

15. Marmot M, Wilkinson RG, eds. *Social Determinants of Health.* Oxford: Oxford University Press; 1999.

16. Wilkinson R, Marmot M, eds. *Social Determinants of Health: The Solid Facts.* 2nd ed. Geneva: World Health Organization; 2003.

17. Marmot M. Social determinants of health inequalities. *Lancet.* 2005; 365:1099–1104.

18. Commission on Social Determinants of Health. *Closing the Gap in a Generation: Health Equity through Action on the Social Determinants of Health. Final Report of the Commission on Social Determinants of Health.* Geneva: World Health Organization; 2008.

19. The John D. and Catherine T. MacArthur Foundation Research Network on Socioeconomic Status and Health. *Reaching for a Healthier Life: Facts on Socioeconomic Status and Health in the United States.* Chicago: John D. and Catherine T. MacArthur Foundation Research Network on Socioeconomic Status and Health; 2008. http://www.macses.ucsf.edu/downloads/Reaching_for_a_Healthier_Life.pdf. Accessed March 28, 2010.

20. Braveman PA, Cubbin C, Egerter S, Williams DR, Pamuk E. Socioeconomic disparities in health in the United States: What the patterns tell us. *Am J Public Health.* 2010;100(Suppl 1):S186–S196.

21. Braveman P, Egerter S, Williams D. Social determinants of health: Coming of age. *Annu Rev Public Health.* 2011;32:381–398.

22. Woolf SH, Dekker MM, Byrne FR, Miller WD. Citizen-centered health promotion: Building collaborations to facilitate healthy living. *Am J Prev Med.* 2011;40(1 Suppl 1):S38–S47.

23. Frieden TR. A framework for public health action: The health impact pyramid. *Am J Public Health.* 2010;100:590–595.

24. Link BG, Phelan J. Social conditions as fundamental causes of disease. *J Health Soc Behav.* 1995;35(extra issue):80–94.

25. Adler NE, Stewart J. Health disparities across the lifespan: Meaning, methods and mechanisms. *Ann N Y Acad Sci.* 2010;1186:5–23.

26. Institute of Medicine. *The Future of the Public's Health in the 21st Century.* Washington, DC: National Academies Press; 2002.

27. Braveman P, Egerter S. *Overcoming Obstacles to Health.* Princeton, NJ: Robert Wood Johnson Foundation Commission to Build a Healthier America; 2008.

28. Marmot MG, Smith GD, Stansfeld S, et al. Health inequalities among British civil servants: The Whitehall II study. *Lancet.* 1991;337(8754):1387–1393.

29. Adams PF, Barnes PM, Vickerie JL. Summary health statistics for the U.S. population: National Health Interview Survey, 2007. National Center for Health Statistics. *Vital Health Stat.* 2008;10(238).

30. Krieger N, Rehkopf DH, Chen JT, Waterman PD, Marcelli E, Kennedy M.

The fall and rise of U.S. inequities in premature mortality: 1960–2002. *PLoS Med.* 2008;5:e46.

31. Woolf SH, Jones RM, Johnson RE, Phillips RL Jr, Oliver MN, Vichare A. Avertable deaths associated with household income in Virginia. *Am J Public Health.* 2010;100:750–755.

32. Muennig P, Fiscella K, Tancredi D, Franks P. The relative health burden of selected social and behavioral risk factors in the United States: Implications for policy. *Am J Public Health.* 2010;100:1758–1764.

33. Project on Societal Distress. Virginia Commonwealth University Center on Human Needs. http://www.societaldistress.org/.

34. Elo IT, Preston SH. Educational differentials in mortality: United States, 1979–85. *Soc Sci Med.* 1996;42:47–57.

35. Jemal A, Thun MJ, Ward EE, Henley SJ, Cokkinides VE, Murray TE. Mortality from leading causes by education and race in the United States, 2001. *Am J Prev Med.* 2008;34:1–8.

36. Woolf SH, Johnson RE, Phillips RL Jr, Philipsen M. Giving everyone the health of the educated: An examination of whether social change would save more lives than medical advances. *Am J Public Health.* 2007;97:679–683.

37. DeNavas-Walt C, Proctor BD, Smith JC. *Income, Poverty, and Health Insurance Coverage in the United States: 2009.* U.S. Census Bureau, Current Population Reports. Washington, DC: U.S. Government Printing Office; 2010.

38. Taylor P, Kochhar R, Fry R, Velasco G, Motel S. *Wealth Gaps Rise to Record Highs between Whites, Blacks and Hispanics.* Washington, DC: Pew Research Center; 2011.

39. Adler NE, Rehkopf DH. U.S. disparities in health: Descriptions, causes, and mechanisms. *Annu Rev Public Health.* 2008;29:235–252.

40. Kawachi I, Adler NE, Dow WH. Money, schooling, and health: Mechanisms and causal evidence. *Ann N Y Acad Sci.* 2010;1186:56–68.

41. Appendix A. Models of health determinants. In: *The Future of the Public's Health in the 21st Century.* Committee on Assuring the Health of the Public in the 21st Century, Board on Health Promotion and Disease Prevention. Washington, DC: National Academies Press; 2002: 401–405.

42. Braveman PA, Egerter SA, Mockenhaupt RE. Broadening the focus: The need to address the social determinants of health. *Am J Prev Med.* 2011;40(1 Suppl 1):S4–S18.

43. Lynch JW, Kaplan GA, Salonen JT. Why do poor people behave poorly? Variation in adult health behaviours and psychosocial characteristics by stages of the socioeconomic lifecourse. *Soc Sci Med.* 1997;44:809–819.

44. Droomers M, Schrijvers CT, Mackenbach JP. Educational level and decreases in leisure time physical activity: Predictors from the longitudinal GLOBE study. *J Epidemiol Community Health.* 2001;55:562–568.

45. Stringhini S, Sabia S, Shipley M, Brunner E, Nabi H, Kivimaki M, Singh-Manoux A. Association of socioeconomic position with health behaviors and mortality. *JAMA.* 2010;303(12):1159–1166.

46. Dunn JR. Health behavior vs the stress of low socioeconomic status and health outcomes. *JAMA.* 2010;303(12):1159–1200.

47. Rod NH, Grønbaek M, Schnohr P, Prescott E, Kristensen TS. Perceived stress as a risk factor for changes in health behaviour and cardiac risk profile: A longitudinal study. *J Intern Med.* 2009;266:467–475.

48. Umberson D, Liu H, Reczek C. Stress and health behaviour over the life course. *Adv Life Course Res.* 2008;13:19–44.

49. Brownell KD, Kersh R, Ludwig DS, Post RC, Puhl RM, Schwartz MB, Willett WC. Personal responsibility and obesity: A constructive approach to a controversial issue. *Health Aff.* 2010;29(3):379–387.

50. Larson NI, Story MT, Nelson MC. Neighborhood environments: Disparities in access to healthy foods in the U.S. *Am J Prev Med.* 2009;36:74–81.

51. Moore LV, Diez Roux AV, Nettleton JA, Jacobs DR. Associations of the local food environment with diet quality—a comparison of assessments based on surveys and geographic information systems: The multi-ethnic study of atherosclerosis. *Am J Epidemiol.* 2008;167(8):917–924.

52. Morland K, Wing S, Roux AD. The contextual effect of the local food environment on residents' diets: The Atherosclerosis Risk in Communities Study. *Am J Public Health.* 2002;92(11):1761–1768.

53. Morland K, Diez Roux AV, Wing S. Supermarkets, other food stores, and obesity: The Atherosclerosis Risk in Communities Study. *Am J Prev Med.* 2006;30(4):333–339.

54. Powell LM, Slater S, Mirtcheva D, Bao Y, Chaloupka FJ. Food store availability and neighborhood characteristics in the United States. *Prev Med.* 2007;44:189–195.

55. Treuhaft S, Karpyn A. *The Grocery Gap: Who Has Access to Healthy Food and Why It Matters.* Oakland, CA: PolicyLink; 2010.

56. Kwate NO, Yau CY, Loh JM, Williams D. Inequality in obesigenic environments: Fast food density in New York City. *Health Place.* 2009;15:364–373.

57. National Cancer Institute. *The Role of the Media in Promoting and Reducing Tobacco Use.* Tobacco Control Monograph No. 19. NIH Pub. No. 07-6242. Bethesda, MD: U.S. Department of Health and Human Services, National Institutes of Health, National Cancer Institute; June 2008.

58. Small ML, McDermott M. The presence of organizational resources in poor urban neighborhoods: An analysis of average and contextual effects. *Social Forces.* 2006;84:1697–1724.

59. Wechsler H, Brener N, Kuester S, Miller C. Food service and foods and beverages available at school: Results from the School Health Policies and Programs Study 2000. *J Sch Health.* 2001;71:313–324.

60. Boone-Heinonen J, Diez Roux AV, Kiefe CI, Lewis CE, Guilkey DK, Gordon-Larsen P. Neighborhood socioeconomic status predictors of physical activity through young to middle adulthood: The CARDIA study. *Soc Sci Med.* 2011;72:641–649.

61. Lynch JW, Kaplan GA, Salonen JT. Why do poor people behave poorly? Variation in adult health behaviours and psychosocial characteristics by stages of the socioeconomic lifecourse. *Soc Sci Med.* 1997;44:809–819.

62. Stringhini S, Dugravot A, Shipley M, Goldberg M, Zins M, Kivimäki M, Marmot M, Sabia S, Singh-Manoux A. Health behaviours, socioeconomic status, and mortality: Further analyses of the British Whitehall II and the French GAZEL prospective cohorts. *PLoS Med.* 2011;8(2):e1000419.

63. Lantz PM, House JS, Lepkowski JM, Williams DR, Mero RP, Chen J. Socioeconomic factors, health behaviors, and mortality: Results from a nationally representative prospective study of U.S. adults. *JAMA*. 1998;279:1703–1708.

64. Diez-Roux AV, Nieto FJ, Muntaner C, Tyroler HA, Comstock GW, Shahar E, Cooper LS, Watson RL, Szklo M. Neighborhood environments and coronary heart disease: A multilevel analysis. *Am J Epidemiol*. 1997;146:48–63.

65. Robert SA. Socioeconomic position and health: The independent contribution of community socioeconomic context. *Annu Rev Sociol*. 1999;25:489–516.

66. Sampson RJ, Morenoff JD, Gannon RT. Assessing "neighborhood effects": Social processes and new directions in research. *Annu Rev Sociol*. 2002;28:443–478.

67. Brulle RJ, Pellow DN. Environmental justice: Human health and environmental inequalities. *Annu Rev Public Health*. 2006;27:103–124.

68. Mohai P, Lantz PM, Morenoff J, House JS, Mero RP. Racial and socioeconomic disparities in residential proximity to polluting industrial facilities: Evidence from the Americans' Changing Lives Study. *Am J Public Health*. 2009;99(Suppl 3):S649–S656.

69. Fujiwara T, Kawachi I. A study of adult twins in the U.S. *Ann N Y Acad Sci*. 2010;1186:139–144.

70. Berkman L, Kawachi I. *Social Epidemiology*. Oxford: Oxford University Press; 2000.

71. Primack BA, Bost JE, Land SR, Fine MJ. Volume of tobacco advertising in African American markets: Systematic review and meta-analysis. *Public Health Rep*. 2007;122(5):607–615.

72. Kwate NO, Meyer IH. Association between residential exposure to outdoor alcohol advertising and problem drinking among African American women in New York City. *Am J Public Health*. 2009;99:228–230.

73. John R, Cheney MK, Azad MR. Point-of-sale marketing of tobacco products: Taking advantage of the socially disadvantaged? *J Health Care Poor Underserved*. 2009;20(2):489–506.

74. Grier SA, Kumanyika SK. The context for choice: Health implications of targeted food and beverage marketing to African Americans. *Am J Public Health*. 2008;98(9):1616–1629.

75. Williams DR, Collins C. Racial residential segregation: A fundamental cause of racial disparities in health. *Public Health Rep*. 2001;116(5):404–416.

76. Schulz AJ, Williams DR, Israel BA, Lempert LB. Racial and spatial relations as fundamental determinants of health in Detroit. *Milbank Q*. 2002;80(4):677–707.

77. Subramanian SV, Acevedo-Garcia D, Osypuk TL. Racial residential segregation and geographic heterogeneity in black/white disparity in poor self-rated health in the U.S.: A multilevel statistical analysis. *Soc Sci Med*. 2005;60:1667–1679.

78. Richardson LD, Norris M. Access to health and health care: How race and ethnicity matter. *Mt Sinai J Med*. 2010;77:166–177.

79. Do DP, Finch BK, Basurto-Davila R, Bird C, Escarce J, Lurie N. Does place explain racial health disparities? Quantifying the contribution of residential context to the black/white health gap in the United States. *Soc Sci Med*. 2008;67(8):1258–1268.

80. Williams DR, Mohammed SA. Discrimination and racial disparities in health: Evidence and needed research. *J Behav Med*. 2009;32:20–47.

81. Jargowsky PA. *Poverty and Place: Ghettos, Barrios and the American City.* New York: Russell Sage Foundation; 1997.

82. Harrington M. *The Other America: Poverty in the United States.* New York: Touchstone; 1997.

83. Charles CA. The dynamics of racial residential segregation. *Annu Rev Sociol.* 2003;29:167–207.

84. Galea S, Tracy M, Hoggatt KJ, Dimaggio C, Karpati A. Estimated deaths attributable to social factors in the United States. *Am J Public Health.* 2011;101:1456–1465.

85. McKewen B, Gianaros PJ. Central role of the brain in stress and adaptation: Links to socioeconomic status, health, and disease. *Ann N Y Acad Sci.* 2010;1186:190–222.

86. Cohen S, Janicki-Deverts D, Chen E, Matthews KA. Childhood socioeconomic status and adult health. *Ann N Y Acad Sci.* 2010;1186:37–55.

87. Fiscella K. Does prenatal care improve birth outcomes? A critical review. *Obstet Gynecol.* 1995;85:468–479.

88. Daniels N, Kennedy B, Kawachi I. *Is Inequality Bad for Our Health?* Boston: Beacon Press; 2000.

89. Wilkinson R, Pickett K. *The Spirit Level: Why Greater Equality Makes Societies Stronger.* New York: Bloomsbury Press; 2009.

90. Organization for Economic Cooperation and Development. OECD Health Data 2011. Health status (mortality) table. http://www.oecd.org/dataoecd/52/42/48304068 .xls#'LE Totalpopulationatbirth'!A1. Accessed August 16, 2011.

91. National Center for Health Statistics. *Health, United States, 2007 with Chartbook on Trends in the Health of Americans.* Hyattsville, MD: 2007. Table 25: Infant mortality rates and international rankings: Selected countries and territories selected years 1960–2004. http://www.cdc.gov/nchs/data/hus/hus07.pdf#025. Accessed September 6, 2011.

92. Crimmins E, Preston SH, Cohen B, eds. *Explaining Divergent Levels of Longevity in High-Income Countries.* Washington, DC: National Academies Press; 2011.

93. Starfield B, Shi L. Policy relevant determinants of health: An international perspective. *Health Policy.* 2002;60:201–218.

94. UNICEF. *Child Poverty in Perspective: An Overview of Child Well-Being in Rich Countries.* Innocenti Report Card 7, 2007 UNICEF Innocenti Research Centre. Florence: United Nations Children's Fund; 2007.

95. Avendano M, Kawachi I. Invited commentary: The search for explanations of the American health disadvantage relative to the English. *Am J Epidemiol.* 2011;173:866–869.

96. Dow WH, Rehkopf DH. Socioeconomic gradients in health in international and historical context. *Ann N Y Acad Sci.* 2010;1186:24–36.

97. Zaza S, Briss PA, Harris KW, eds. *The Guide to Community Preventive Services: What Works to Promote Health?* New York: Oxford University Press; 2005.

98. Wasserman J, Manning WG, Newhouse JP, Winkler JD. The effects of excise taxes and regulations on cigarette smoking. *J Health Econ.* 1991;10:43–64.

99. Levy DT, Chaloupka F, Gitchell J. The effects of tobacco control policies on smoking rates: A tobacco control scorecard. *J Public Health Manag Pract.* 2004;10:338–353.

100. Frieden TR, Bassett MT, Thorpe LE, Farley TA. Public health in New

York City, 2002–2007: Confronting epidemics of the modern era. *Int J Epidemiol.* 2008;37:966–977.

101. Frieden TR, Bloomberg MR. How to prevent 100 million deaths from tobacco. *Lancet.* 2007;369(9574):1758–1761.

102. Brownson RC, Haire-Joshu D, Luke DA. Shaping the context of health: A review of environmental and policy approaches in the prevention of chronic diseases. *Annu Rev Public Health.* 2006;27:341–370.

103. Collins J, Koplan JP. Health impact assessment: A step toward health in all policies. *JAMA.* 2009;302(3):315–317.

104. Cole BL, Fielding JE. Health impact assessment: A tool to help policy makers understand health beyond health care. *Annu Rev Public Health.* 2007;28:393–412.

105. Dannenberg AL, Bhatia R, Cole BL, Heaton SK, Feldman JD, Rutt CD. Use of health impact assessment in the U.S.: 27 case studies, 1999–2007. *Am J Prev Med.* 2008;34(3):241–256.

106. Strategic Growth Council. Health in All Policies Task Force. Sacramento, CA: Strategic Growth Council. http://www.sgc.ca.gov/hiap/. Accessed April 1, 2011.

107. National Prevention, Health Promotion, and Public Health Council. 2010 Annual Status Report. Washington, DC: Department of Health and Human Services; July 1, 2010. http://www.hhs.gov/news/reports/nationalprevention2010report.pdf. Accessed April 1, 2011.

108. Miller W, Simon P, Maleque S. *Beyond Health Care: New Directions to a Healthier America.* Washington, DC: Robert Wood Johnson Foundation Commission to Build a Healthier America; 2009.

109. Institute of Medicine. *For the Public's Health: The Role of Measurement in Action and Accountability.* Washington, DC: National Academies Press; 2011.

110. *Unnatural Causes* (documentary film). http://www.unnaturalcauses.org/.

2

The Health of Marginalized Populations

Richard Ingram, Julia F. Costich, and Debra Joy Pérez

The United States: Pockets of Health Inequity

The health status of the United States as a whole can be described as reasonably poor relative to other industrial nations. Evidence suggests that, while the United States ranks first among all countries in health care spending, it ranks thirty-sixth in life expectancy, thirty-ninth in infant mortality, forty-second in adult male mortality, and forty-third in adult female mortality.[1] This may be due, at least in part, to an underperforming health care system; the U.S. health care system performs poorly when compared with other nations, ranking last or next to last in quality, access, efficiency, equity, and healthy lives while ranking first, again, in terms of cost.[2] These statistics, though compelling, do not tell the entire story. The comparatively poor health of the United States is just one symptom of a deeper problem: health inequity. The United States is rife with pockets of both good health, where citizens have access to excellent health care and a large share of the nation's plenty, and poor health, where citizens are marginalized economically and educationally and do not have access to their fair share of the nation's wealth or to good health care.

Sharp differences in health status exist among individual states. *America's Health Rankings*, released by the United Health Foundation, measures states' status in areas such as health behaviors, community and environmental factors, public and health policies, clinical care, and health outcomes.[3] The 2010 edition of the rankings found that citizens of Vermont enjoyed the highest health status, with an average health score 1.131 standard deviations above the mean U.S. score. In contrast, citizens of Mississippi suffered the worst health, with an average health score –0.786 standard deviations below the mean.[3]

When viewed at any level, geography may explain some of the health differences between and among populations, but it does not explain all of them. There appear to be sharp inequities between Mississippi and Vermont with regard to the socioecological determinants of health and health status. Vermont has less poverty: 12 percent of the children in Vermont live at or below the poverty threshold, compared with 31.9 percent of Mississippi's children.[3] Vermont does a better job educating its children, with approximately 88.6 percent of incoming ninth graders graduating from high school in four years; in Mississippi, this number drops to 63.6 percent.[3] It should therefore be no surprise that per capita personal income is $38,503 in Vermont and only $30,103 in Mississippi.[3] Income is also distributed more equitably in Vermont: the Gini coefficient (a measure of income inequality, where a value of 0 indicates complete equality and a value of 1 complete inequality) is 0.434 for Vermont and 0.478 for Mississippi.[3]

Inequities do not exist just between states; they exist within them as well. Each year, the University of Wisconsin Population Health Institute, with support from the Robert Wood Johnson Foundation, calculates the County Health Rankings, a measure of the health status (including mortality, morbidity, health behaviors, clinical care, social and economic factors, and physical environment) of all counties in the United States relative to their peers in each state.[4] The rankings show that the citizens of some counties enjoy far greater access to the socioecological determinants of health and greater health status than do citizens in other counties in the same state. For example, the 2011 edition of the rankings found that even within Vermont (the healthiest state, according to *America's Health Rankings*), the smoking rate in Essex County (30 percent) was more than double that in Chittenden County (14 percent).[4] Access to health care also varied widely between the two counties. While Essex County's ratio of population to primary care physicians was 1,292:1, Chittenden County had a much more favorable ratio of 306:1.[4]

There were also sharp differences in the socioecological determinants of health between Chittenden and Essex Counties. Nine percent of the children in Chittenden County lived at or below the poverty level, versus 24 percent of the children in Essex County.[4] Chittenden County's unemployment rate was 5.9 percent, compared with 9.2 percent in Essex County.[4] These stark economic differences were manifested at school, where 55.1 percent of students in Essex County received subsidized school lunches in 2010, but only 26.5 percent of students in Chittenden County did so.[5]

Marginalized Populations: Common Cultures, Uncommonly Poor Health

Similar pockets of health inequity exist throughout the United States. Although these pockets are often categorized as discrete geographic units, they share more than geography. They are often culturally distinct, enjoying a rich and unique identity. However, they share one commonality: the people inside their boundaries have been marginalized by society. The marginalization of these populations manifests itself in many ways. The people in these areas do not have access to the same levels of high-quality education as their neighbors. They do not have access to the same levels of income as their neighbors and thus experience greater poverty. As a result, they often have much less access to health care resources and poorer health than their neighbors. They have neither the health nor the wealth to take full advantage of the nation's resources.

Marginalized populations often do not fit into tidy geographic boundaries. They may occupy a multistate region, an entire state, multiple counties within a state, or sometimes only a particular neighborhood. Specific examples of marginalized populations characterized by economic, educational, and health inequities are the multistate Appalachian region of the United States, the state of Kentucky, Alabama's "Black Belt," and the Barrio Logan neighborhood of San Diego. These are just four examples of the extreme inequities and socioecological factors that contribute to disparities in health and health care.

Appalachia

Economy, poverty, and education in Appalachia

It is impossible to understand the health status of the people of Appalachia or any other marginalized population without first understanding the disparities in the underlying causes of health—particularly income, poverty, and education—experienced by that population. The Appalachian region roughly follows the spine of the Appalachian mountain range from southern New York to northern Mississippi.[6] It encompasses over 205,000 square miles and is made up of 420 counties in thirteen states. It is home to 24.8 million people,[6,7] and its residents are overwhelmingly white.[8] Appalachia is characterized by a mountainous, rugged landscape. As a result, the people in Appalachia are two times more likely than other Americans to live in rural areas: 42 percent of Appalachians live in rural areas, compared with only 20 percent of the total U.S. population.[6] The residents of Appalachia are, on average, older, poorer, less educated, and less healthy than the nation as a whole.[6,7,9]

Wealth is a key determinant of health, and residents of Appalachia do not have access to the same financial resources as the rest of the United States. The regional economy has diversified in recent times, focusing less on resource extraction, chemical manufacturing, and heavy industry.[6,7] Although this has led to economic gains in the region, individual income still lags behind that in the rest of the nation. In 2008 the average per capita income in Appalachia was $32,411, almost 20 percent less than the national average of $40,166. This income disparity is even wider when looked at from the context of market income (a measure that doesn't factor in transfer payments), in which case the 2008 per capita income in Appalachia was more than 25 percent less than the national average.[7]

One result of the economic inequity between Appalachia and the rest of United States is that the region has higher rates of poverty, another key determinant of health. Appalachia is less poor than it once was, but the average poverty rate in Appalachia in 2005–2009 was 15.4 percent, while the U.S. average was 13.5 percent.[10] Although this may not seem to be a significant disparity, a sizable number of marginally poor areas skewed the average poverty rate toward the mean, thus obscuring a large number of counties in the region, concentrated mainly in Kentucky, with poverty rates exceeding 25 percent.[7, 10]

Education can be a passport to a better life, higher earnings, and better health, and lack of educational attainment can be a major cause of poor health. In 2000 Appalachia had a lower average high school completion rate (76.8 percent) than the U.S. average (80.4 percent).[7] Once again, this disparity may not seem great, but as with the poverty rate, a large number of counties with graduation rates closer to the national average (around 61 to 76 percent) obscured the many counties, once again in Kentucky, with rates less than 61 percent.[7] The disparity in college completion rates in 2000 was even greater: 17.6 percent of Appalachians had completed college, compared with a national average of 24.4 percent.[7]

The health of Appalachia

Given these bleak statistics, it should come as no surprise that there are serious health inequities between Appalachia and the nation as a whole. Evidence suggests that residents of Appalachian areas have higher rates of health risks such as smoking, adiposity, and hypertension.[11] These areas also have higher levels of socioeconomic inequality.[12-14] Behavior and socioeconomic conditions combine to cause a cascade of health challenges that contribute to the fact that Appalachia experiences much higher rates of premature mortality related to certain conditions compared with the rest of the nation.[12-14] Those living in Appalachia have a higher incidence of various cancers than those living in other parts of the United States.[13, 15-17] The incidence of diabetes in Appalachia exceeds the incidence in the rest of the nation,[13, 14, 18, 19] and there are much higher rates of diseases related to diabetes, including heart disease and stroke.[11, 13, 18, 20, 21]

Kentucky

Economy, poverty, and education in Kentucky

Kentucky is one of the thirteen states in Appalachia. Its topography is fairly diverse, ranging from the steep mountains and hills in the eastern (Appalachian) part of the state to the rolling fields of the Bluegrass region in the center of the state. It encompasses 40,407.80 square miles, making it the thirty-seventh largest state.[22] In 2009 it had a population of approximately 4,314,113, making it the twenty-sixth most populous state.[23] The majority of Kentucky's residents are white.[24] The 2000 census showed that a slim majority of Kentuckians lived in urban areas; however, the 2010 census indicated a dramatic migration from rural to urban areas in Kentucky, resulting in a steep decline in the rural population.[25]

Kentucky is a relatively poor state, with a per capita income in 2011 of approximately $32,376 (ranking forty-seventh out of the fifty states). It fares marginally better when analyzed in terms of income equity, ranking thirty-seventh and having a Gini coefficient of 0.466.[3] Kentucky experiences much greater levels of poverty than most other states. It ranks forty-second (tied with three other states) in the percentage of children living in poverty (26 percent) and is tied for forty-fifth (with four other states) in terms of the proportion of the population living under the poverty level (19 percent).[5] The economic prospects of Kentuckians are furthered dimmed by the relatively low high school graduation rate: 74.4 percent, placing it thirty-second among the fifty states.[3]

The health of Kentucky

Given the wide gulf between the state and the rest of the country with regard to economic conditions, poverty, and education, it is no surprise that Kentucky ranks poorly in many measures of health. When it comes to premature deaths, it ranks forty-second (fiftieth being the worst).[3] Like in the nation as a whole, heart disease and cancer are the leading causes of death among Kentuckians, but they seem to suffer an undue burden of these diseases.[26] Kentucky ranks forty-seventh in the percentage of adults who have had heart attacks, fiftieth in cancer death rates, and thirty-eighth in the percentage of adults with diabetes.[3] Cancer has recently overtaken heart disease as the most common cause of death among Kentucky women when data are adjusted for age, while heart disease remains the most common cause of death in the absence of age adjustment.[27] There are stark racial inequities in Kentucky: African American Kentuckians die earlier and have higher death rates from both heart disease and cancer, as well as from cerebrovascular disease and diabetes mellitus, but they have lower death rates from suicide, pneumonia, and renal failure.

Like in Vermont and Mississippi, Kentucky's statewide totals mask tremendous intrastate variation, due in part to the migration of relative young and healthy residents from certain areas. With regard to overall death rates, the county with the highest age-adjusted rate (Owsley, 1,293.9 per 100,000) is 58 percent higher than the county at the other extreme (Calloway, 817 per 100,000). Even more striking, the age-adjusted death rate from lung cancer in Perry County is 282 percent that of Washington County.

Kentucky's poor health status results in a tremendous but difficult to quantify burden of disease. For example, the cost of cardiovascular-related hospitalization in Kentucky was estimated to be $2.2 billion in 2005, while the cost of diabetes was estimated at $2.9 million in 2002.[28, 29] An indirect measure of Kentucky's disease burden is the proportion of a county's under-65 population covered by Medicare. To qualify for Medicare coverage, individuals younger than 65 must be seriously work-disabled. Overall, 4.7 percent of the state's residents fall into this category, but countywide percentages range from more than 10 percent in Pike, Harlan, Leslie, Floyd, Perry, and Webster Counties to less than 2 percent in Whitley and Oldham Counties. These Medicare data suggest that the burden of ill health is concentrated in counties that have lost substantial numbers of able-bodied working-age adults, leaving their populations increasingly elderly and disabled.

Medicare patients are more likely than other Kentuckians to be hospitalized, but it is nonetheless striking how frequently Kentucky Medicare beneficiaries use inpatient services compared with national norms: they are well above the 90th percentile for both number of inpatient stays (406.3 per 1,000 beneficiaries) and number of inpatient days per beneficiary.[30] Notably, onefourth of inpatient stays (103.5 per 1,000) were for conditions that, at least arguably, could have been treated in an ambulatory care setting if they had been managed appropriately on an outpatient basis. Whether these figures represent overuse or an unusually high burden of disease is debatable, but there is no question that they add to the cost of care, averaging $8,518 per Medicare beneficiary in 2007, the most recent year for which data have been reported.

Kentucky's relatively poor performances with regard to health and the economy combine to create a self-reinforcing negative feedback loop that makes it exponentially more difficult for the state to improve in either area. There is growing evidence that social determinants are major factors in health status. Lindstrom summarizes current knowledge in this area: "The association between social circumstances and health-related behaviors is now widely accepted as a major health determinant. The social environment affects individual health-related behavior through a number of causal mechanisms by shaping

Table 2.1. Education, Poverty, and Health Status by County Health Rankings Quartile

Quartile	Percentage of High School Graduates	Percentage in Poverty
1st	76.7	15.1
2nd	69.7	19.3
3rd	66.9	20.2
4th	57.3	30.9

Source: County Health Rankings: Mobilizing Action toward Community Health. 2011. http//www.countyhealthrankings.org

norms, enforcing social control, enabling or not enabling people to participate in particular behaviors, reducing or producing stress, and constraining individual choice."[31] One example of the link between health and the economy is Kentucky's high rate of childhood overweight and obesity (34.4 percent).[6] Although being overweight clearly predisposes children to unhealthy adult lives, the prevalence of overweight and obesity has also been considered as a factor in business location decision making. Thus, the high prevalence of childhood overweight and obesity not only puts the state at risk for increased health care costs but also denies it the necessary resources to combat the effects of these conditions through increased economic development.

The relationships between health status and poverty (as defined by the percentage of the population living in poverty) and health status and education (as defined by high school graduation rates), two common metrics for social determinants, are illustrated in table 2.1. A comparison of four quartiles of health status, as defined by the 2011 County Health Rankings, show that poverty and low educational attainment are directly related to poor health status.[4] The average proportion of county populations over age 25 who have graduated from high school is one-third higher in the healthiest quartile than in the least healthy quartile, and the average poverty rate in the lowest-ranking counties is more than double that of the highest-ranking group.

Alabama's "Black Belt"

Economy, poverty, and education in the Black Belt

Historically, Alabama's so-called Black Belt stretched across seventeen counties in the southern portion of the state, starting on the western border in Sumter and Choctaw Counties and ending at Russell and Barbour Counties on the eastern border.[32] It now encompasses only twelve counties, starting in the same western counties but now ending in Bullock and Macon Counties near the southern border.[33] It is heavily forested and is characterized by rich, black loamy soil. Like Appalachia, it is heavily rural and sparsely populated. The 2006 population of the Black Belt was approximately 212,148, a small proportion of Alabama's total population of 4,599,030 people.[33] Sixty-four percent of the Black Belt's population was black in 2006, compared with 24 percent for the rest of the state.[33, 34] The region holds an average of twenty-three people per square mile. However, this number is deceiving, as it drops sharply to three people per square mile outside of the few cities in the region.[35] The residents of the Black Belt are, on average, older, poorer, less educated, and less healthy than residents of Alabama as a whole.

The residents of the Black Belt, similar to the residents of Appalachia, do not have access to the same financial resources as the rest of Alabama. The regional economy at one time depended heavily on cotton farming; currently it depends on timber production. The largest landowners in each of the Black Belt counties are timber producers, and most of that land is owned by entities located outside county lines.[35] Timber companies enjoy tax rates far lower than those imposed on other industries. As a result, the tax base of the Black Belt counties is lower than that in much of the state, making it difficult to fund basic services such as education.[35] The jobs available to residents of the Black Belt do not pay well; in 2005 the average per capita income in the region was $22,406, more than 25 percent lower than the Alabama average of $29,623.[33]

The economic inequities in the region manifest themselves in high poverty rates. In 2004, 16.1 percent of the population of Alabama lived in poverty, but the poverty rate in the Black Belt was more than 50 percent higher, at 25.7 percent.[33] Thirty-seven percent of households in the Black Belt earn less than $15,000 a year—more than twice the U.S. rate.[35]

Residents of the Black Belt also face inequities in education. While the high school graduation rate for the state of Alabama as a whole was 61.7 percent, the graduation rate for the counties in the Black Belt was only 59.3 percent. Once again, this seemingly insignificant difference, based on averages, hides the poor performance of four counties in the region with rates at or below 55 percent.[5] During the six-year period from 1996 through 2001, the Black Belt contained eight of the ten lowest-scoring school systems on the Stanford Achievement Test; the average score in Black Belt schools was 41.5, while the state average was 55.7.[36] The severe poverty of the region also manifests itself at school, where more than 80 percent of students qualified for free and reduced-cost lunches during 1999 and 2000; only 44 percent of students in the rest of the state qualified for the program.[36]

The health of the Black Belt

Given the severe inequities in earnings, poverty, and education in the Black Belt compared with the rest of Alabama, it is no surprise that inequities in health exist as well. These inequities start in the womb. In 2003–2005, 33.5 percent of births in the Black Belt were to mothers who had not received adequate prenatal care, while the state average was 23.1 percent.[33] In 1997 some Black Belt counties had life expectancies less than those of developing nations such as Sri Lanka, Ecuador, and El Salvador.[34] Residents of the region experience much higher total rates of cancer, as well as cancers of the digestive tract and prostate, than the state as a whole. In 2003–2005 statewide diabetes rates were more than 25 percent less than those in the Black Belt, heart disease rates were more than 33 percent lower, and stroke rates were considerably lower as well. The inequities experienced by residents of the Black Belt persist until death. In 2005 life expectancy in the counties making up the Black Belt was 72.9 years, less than the state average of 74.8 years.[33]

Barrio Logan

Economy, poverty, and education in Barrio Logan

The Barrio Logan neighborhood is located in the southeastern part of San Diego, California. In 2000 Barrio Logan was home to 3,636 people, 86 percent of whom were Hispanic.[37] Much of the neighborhood lies along the Pacific coast and is home to Chicano Park, an idyllic setting characterized by a rich abundance of art and events that celebrate Chicano culture.

Barrio Logan is an urban, industrial area with heavy port traffic.[38, 39] The community is exposed to approximately 3 million pounds of toxic air pollutants released each year.[39] Because it is a major shipping area, residents are exposed to high levels of diesel exhaust and particulate matter.[38, 40] Barrio Logan is home to more than 384 sites that pollute, generate hazardous waste, or handle chemicals, and it is in close proximity to another 275 potentially toxic sites.[41] Residents of the area are exposed to high levels of toxic chemicals such as hydrocarbons, hexavalent chromium, and lead.[41]

Although the profusion of industry in Barrio Logan has brought pollution, it has brought neither wealth nor jobs to the area. In 1999, 49 percent of households reported incomes of less than $20,000.[37] According to the 2000 census, of the 2,376 individuals aged 16 or older living in the neighborhood, only 1,207 were employed.[37] As a result, the health of the residents of Barrio Logan is threatened by poverty as well as pollution. According to the 2000 census, approximately 40 percent of the residents of Barrio Logan lived in poverty—much higher than the regional rate of 12.6 percent.[37] Of particular concern is the impact of poverty on children. In 2000, 734 families with children lived in poverty in Barrio Logan; 240 of these families lived below the poverty level. Many families also lived in substandard housing.[39, 40]

The residents of Barrio Logan also experience low educational attainment. According to the 2000 census, only 22 percent of the residents aged 25 and older had obtained a high school diploma or its equivalent. Five percent had obtained an associate's degree, and only 2 percent had obtained a bachelor's degree.[37]

The health of Barrio Logan

The scant evidence that exists suggests that economic, educational, and environmental conditions have a significant impact on the health of Barrio Logan residents, particularly the children. There is evidence that they have unusually high rates of lead poisoning when compared with their peers.[40, 42] The children in the neighborhood also have higher rates of asthma, perhaps related to the extremely polluted air and substandard housing.[38, 42] Finally, low-birth-weight, preterm babies may be more common in the area.[40]

Why Do These Marginalized Populations Exhibit Poor Health?

The clinician's perspective

The reasons for the poorer health status of residents of these four areas compared with their fellow citizens can be viewed from two perspectives. From a strictly clinical perspective, the health inequities experienced by the residents of Appalachia, Kentucky, the Black Belt, Barrio Logan, and other marginalized populations are simply a large-scale manifestation of individual differences in risk factors and risk behaviors.[43] The residents of Appalachia and the Black Belt have inordinate levels of heart disease because they smoke more and have less healthy diets than their peers; the residents of Barrio Logan simply live in the wrong place. The clinical approach to rectifying these disparities focuses on the personal causes of poor health, such as genetics, individual behavior, knowledge, and access, and it focuses largely on improving the delivery of services to individuals.[43, 44]

At first, a clinical approach to eliminating inequity might seem to be a promising means of improving the health of marginalized populations. If inequities are simply the result of too much disease, the simplest and most direct way to eliminate disparities would be to address the individual determinants of disease. Residents of the Black Belt and Appalachia should eat healthier foods and stop smoking; residents of Barrio Logan should move. However, it quickly becomes apparent that such an approach ignores the root causes of disease—socioecological determinants that act to create the inequities manifested in these populations.[43-50]

The socioecological perspective

From a socioecological perspective, the health disparities experienced by marginalized populations are not simply the manifestations of unequal levels of the clinical determinants of health; rather, they are the manifestations of an unequal distribution of the socioecological determinants of health.[43] Disparities in power, money, and the services and goods they buy are seen as the root cause of health disparities.[43-45, 47-49] Given their isolation, the residents of Appalachia and the Black Belt may not be able to afford, or they may not live in close proximity to, the healthy foods and smoking cessation programs available to their peers. The residents of Barrio Logan cannot afford to move. From the socioecological perspective, improving the health of marginalized populations is not simply a matter of improving service delivery or individual behaviors. Rather, the solution is far more complex and is centered on a more equitable access to the socioecological determinants of health.[43, 44, 47, 49, 50] Access to power and wealth, not access to care, may be the key to improving health status.

The inequitable distribution of the socioecological determinants of health is exacerbated by the fact that marginalized populations often feel that they have far less power than their numbers would suggest. As a result, they may believe that they lack the ability to change their situation. A unique phenomenon in American society is that those who have power often receive much greater benefits relative to their need and numbers, while those who lack power receive much lower benefits relative to their need and numbers.[51] This may seem counterintuitive, but it is simply the result of the democratic processes of the United States: policy makers cater to those who will determine their electoral fates. Marginalized populations are often negatively categorized as "weak" or "undeserving."[51] Racism and related issues, such as residential segregation, also play a role in characterizing some citizens as "undeserving" of benefits.[49, 50] Thus, the electorate may view programs that benefit certain populations in a negative light. In addition, marginalized populations may internalize these negative characterizations, causing them to feel powerless; as a result, they may fail to exercise the power they do have.[51]

Crafting a Solution

The root causes of marginalized populations' poor health are complex and multifactorial, and addressing them is not easy. Although attempts to eliminate the disparities experienced by these populations must address access to care, such efforts must target systemic changes that improve the distribution of the socioecological determinants of health.[43, 44, 49] Because marginalized populations often enjoy unique cultures, and because their problems often occur as a result of local factors, effective strategies to address disparities should be rooted in a deep understanding of the community.

Community-based participatory research is one way to engage marginalized populations in research and ensure that such research is culturally sensitive and comprehensive.[38, 39, 52-54] However, this approach comes with potential pitfalls. Community members may perceive such efforts as hierarchical, and researchers may not understand the unique cultures they are studying.[53] One possible solution is to develop, promote, and utilize researchers from marginalized populations, an approach taken by some academic institutions.[52, 55, 56]

The Robert Wood Johnson Foundation (RWJF) has demonstrated an extraordinary commitment to initiatives to facilitate the development of researchers from marginalized populations. One particular effort is the New Connections program, which targets early- to mid-career scholars from historically underrepresented communities in order to increase the diversity of the U.S. professoriat. The program, which has awarded more than 100 grants since its inception in 2006, offers mentoring and research support and strives to increase the diversity of researchers funded by the RWJF and, by extension, the reach and diversity of their research.[57] Another program funded by the RWJF is the Summer Medical and Dental Pipeline. Its goal is to increase the diversity of health services and health policy researchers by providing hundreds of high school students from underrepresented backgrounds with access to methodological training and exposing them to careers in science and medicine.[58] The RWJF also funds the Harold Amos Medical Faculty Development Program, which is intended to increase the number of medical faculty from disadvantaged populations.[59]

Marginalized populations exist in communities throughout the United States. As demonstrated by the examples of Appalachia, Kentucky, the Black Belt, and Barrio Logan, these communities suffer from poorer health compared with their peers, which is simply the manifestation of a deeper systemic problem: inequity in the distribution of the socioecological determinants of health in the United States. Efforts to solve these problems must aim at eliminating systemic inequities if they are to be effective. However, the context of the communities impacted must be considered. These communities are unique and complex, and research and programs targeted at them must both empower and engage their populations.

Notes

1. Murray CJ, Frenk J. Ranking 37th—measuring the performance of the U.S. health care system. *N Engl J Med.* 2010;362(2):98–99.

2. Davis K, Schoen C, Schoenbaum SC, Doty MM, Holmgren AL, Kriss JL, et al. *Mirror, Mirror on the Wall: An International Update on the Comparative Performance of American Health Care.* Report No. 1027. New York: The Commonwealth Fund; 2007.

3. United Health Foundation, Arundel Street Consulting. *America's Health Rankings: A Call to Action for Individuals and Their Communities.* Minnetonka, MN: United Health Foundation; 2010.

4. County Health Rankings: Mobilizing Action toward Community Health. 2011. http://www.countyhealthrankings.org. Accessed October 10, 2011.

5. The Annie E. Casey Foundation Kids Count Data Center. 2011. http://datacenter .kidscount.org. Accessed October 10, 2011.

6. The Appalachian Region. http//www.arc.gov/appalachian_region/The AppalachianRegion.asp. Accessed October 10, 2011.

7. Socioeconomic Overview of Appalachia. 2010. http//www.arc.gov/images/ appregion/SocioeconomicOverviewofAppalachiaMarch2010.pdf. Accessed October 10, 2011.

8. Pollard KM. *A "New Diversity": Race and Ethnicity in the Appalachian Region.* Washington, DC: Appalachian Regional Commission; 2004.

9. Appalachian Regional Commission. *Annual Report.* Washington, DC: Appalachian Regional Commission; 1965.

10. Relative Poverty Rates in Appalachia, 2005–2009. 2011. http://www.arc.gov/ research/MapsofAppalachia.asp?MAP_ID=61. Accessed October 10, 2011.

11. Danaei G, Rimm EB, Oza S, Kulkarni SC, Murray CJL, Ezzati M. The promise of prevention: The effects of four preventable risk factors on national life expectancy and life expectancy disparities by race and county in the United States. *PLoS Med.* 2010;7(3). http:// www.plosmedicine.org/article/info%3Adoi%2F10.1371%2Fjournal.pmed.100024.

12. Behringer B, Friedell GH. Appalachia: Where place matters in health. *Prev Chronic Dis.* 2006;3(4):A113.

13. Halverson JA. *An Analysis of Disparities in Health Status and Access to Care in the Appalachian Region.* Washington, DC: Appalachian Regional Commission; 2004.

14. Halverson JA, Bischak G. *Underlying Socioeconomic Factors Influencing Health Disparities in the Appalachian Region: Final Report.* Washington, DC: Appalachian Regional Commission; 2008.

15. Friedell GH, Tucker TC, McManmon E, Moser M, Hernandez C, Nadel M. Incidence of dysplasia and carcinoma of the uterine cervix in an Applalachian population. *J Natl Cancer Inst.* 1992;84(13):1030–1032.

16. Hall HI, Rogers JD, Weir HK, Miller DS, Uhler RJ. Breast and cervical carcinoma mortality among women in the Appalachian region of the US, 1976–1996. *Cancer.* 2000;89(7):1593–1602.

17. Horner MJ, Altekruse SF, Zou ZH, Wideroff L, Katki HA, Stinchcomb DG. U.S. geographic distribution of prevaccine era cervical cancer screening, incidence, stage, and mortality. *Cancer Epidemiol Biomarkers Prev.* 2011;20(4):591–599.

18. Hendryx M, Zullig KJ. Higher coronary heart disease and heart attack morbidity in Appalachian coal mining regions. *Preventive Med.* 2009;49(5):355–359.

19. Pancoska P, Buch S, Cecchetti A, Parmanto B, Vecchio M, Groark S, et al. Family networks of obesity and type 2 diabetes in rural Appalachia. *Clin Translational Sci.* 2009;2(6):413–421.

20. Hendryx M. Mortality from heart, respiratory, and kidney disease in coal mining areas of Appalachia. *Int Arch Occup Environ Health.* 2009;82(2):243–249.

21. Schwartz F, Ruhil A, Denham S, Shubrook J, Simpson C, Boyd SL. High self-reported prevalence of diabetes mellitus, heart disease, and stroke in 11 counties of rural Appalachian Ohio. *J Rural Health.* 2009;25(2):226–230.

22. U.S. Census Bureau. 2010 Census State Area Measurements and Internal Point Coordinates. http://www.census.gov/geo/www/2010census/statearea_intpt.html. Accessed January 4, 2012.

23. U.S. Census Bureau. State Rankings—Statistical Abstract of the United States, Resident Population—July 2009. http://www.census.gov/compendia/statab/2012/ranks/rank01.html. Accessed January 4, 2012.

24. U.S. Census Bureau. 2010 Population Finder: Kentucky. http://www.census.gov/popfinder/. Accessed January 4, 2012.

25. U.S. Census Bureau. Urban and Rural (6) Universe: Housing Units Census 2000 State Legislative District Summary File (100-Percent). http://factfinder2.census.gov/faces/tableservices/jsf/pages/productview.xhtml?pid=DEC_00_SLDH_H002&prodType=table. Accessed January 4, 2012.

26. Centers for Disease Control and Prevention. CDC Wonder. http://wonder.cdc.gov. Accessed January 4, 2012.

27. Sands H. Preliminary data. Division of Epidemiology, Kentucky Department of Public Health; 2010.

28. Kentucky: Cabinet for Health and Family Services. Kentucky Cardiovascular Disease Fact Sheet. http://chfs.ky.gov/NR/rdonlyres/738A1FCB-4F89–4C25-A6E1–548D3E36BE29/0/KyCVDFactSheet_Aug081.pdf. Accessed January 4, 2012.

29. Kentucky: Cabinet for Health and Family Services. Kentucky Diabetes Fact Sheet 2007. http://chfs.ky.gov/NR/rdonlyres/25F4BA14-D7EF-4DAF-9C50-C2E8E-7AEA0AC/0/DiabetesinKentucky07FS.pdf. Accessed January 4, 2012.

30. Dartmouth Atlas of Health Care. Understanding of the Efficiency and Effectiveness of the Health Care System. http://www.dartmouthatlas.org. Accessed January 4, 2012.

31. Lindstrom M. Social capital and health-related behaviors. In: Kawachi I, Subramanian SV, Kim D, eds. *Social Capital and Health,* citing Institute of Medicine. *The Future of the Public's Health in the 21st Century.* Washington, DC: National Academies Press; 2003.

32. *Traditional Counties of the Alabama Black Belt*. Tuscaloosa: Center for Economic and Business Research at the University of Alabama; 2011.

33. Black Belt Action Commission, Alabama Department of Public Health. Selected Health Status Indicators; 2007.

34. Archibald J, Hansen J. Life is short, prosperity is long gone. *Birmingham News*. May 12, 2002.

35. Archibald J, Hansen J. Land is power, and most who wield it are outsiders. *Birmingham News*. October 13, 2002.

36. Dean CJ, Crowder C, Archibald J. Held back: Poverty hobbling students. *Birmingham News*. October 27, 2002.

37. Census 2000 Profile: Barrio Logan Community Planning Area, City of San Diego. San Diego, CA; June 12, 2003.

38. Hood E. Dwelling disparities: How poor housing leads to poor health. *Environ Health Perspect*. 2005;113(5):A310–A317.

39. Lee C. Environmental justice: Building a unified vision of health and the environment. *Environ Health Perspect*. 2002;110:141–144.

40. English PB, Kharrazi M, Davies S, Scalf R, Waller L, Neutra R. Changes in the spatial pattern of low birth weight in a southern California county: The role of individual and neighborhood level factors. *Soc Sci Med*. 2003;56(10):2073–2088.

41. Ganiere R, Peacock PE. City of San Diego. Environmental data resources (EDR) area study: Barrio Logan. San Diego, CA; 2008.

42. Williams J, Takvorian D, Holmquist S. Environmental Health Coalition. Children at risk? A community based health survey in San Diego's most polluted neighborhoods. National City, CA; 1997.

43. Iton AB. The ethics of the medical model in addressing the root causes of health disparities in local public health practice. *J Public Health Manage Pract*. 2008;14(4):335–339.

44. Green BL, Lewis RK, Bediako SM. Reducing and eliminating health disparities: A targeted approach. *J Natl Med Assoc*. 2005;97(1):25–30.

45. Braveman P. Health disparities and health equity: Concepts and measurement. *Annu Rev Public Health*. 2006;27:167–194.

46. Frist WH. Overcoming disparities in US health care—a broad view of the causes of health disparities can lead to better, more appropriate solutions. *Health Aff*. 2005;24(2):445–451.

47. Graham H. Social determinants and their unequal distribution: Clarifying policy understandings. *Milbank Q*. 2004;82(1):101–124.

48. Olafsdottir S. Fundamental causes of health disparities: Stratification, the welfare state, and health in the United States and Iceland. *J Health Soc Behav*. 2007;48(3):239–253.

49. Shavers VL, Shavers BS. Racism and health inequity among Americans. *J Natl Med Assoc*. 2006;98(3):386–396.

50. Williams DR, Collins C. Racial residential segregation: A fundamental cause of racial disparities in health. *Public Health Rep*. 2001;116(5):404–416.

51. Schneider A, Ingram H. Social construction of target populations: Implications for politics and policy. *Am Polit Sci Rev*. 1993;87(2):334.

52. Viets VL, Baca C, Verney SP, Venner K, Parker T, Wallerstein N. Reducing health disparities through a culturally centered mentorship program for minority faculty: The Southwest Addictions Research Group (SARG) experience. *Acad Med.* 2009;84(8):1118–1126.

53. Arcury TA, Quandt SA, Dearry A. Farmworker pesticide exposure and community-based participation research: Rationale and practical applications. *Environ Health Perspect.* 2001;109:429–434.

54. Quandt SA, Arcury TA, Pell AI. Something for everyone? A community and academic partnership to address farmworker pesticide exposure in North Carolina. *Environ Health Perspect.* 2001;109:435–441.

55. Daley S, Wingard DL, Reznik V. Improving the retention of underrepresented minority faculty in academic medicine. *J Natl Med Assoc.* 2006;98(9):1435–1440.

56. Yager J, Waitzkin H, Parker T, Duran B. Educating, training, and mentoring minority faculty and other trainees in mental health services research. *Acad Psychiatry.* 2007;31(2):146–151.

57. Robert Wood Johnson Foundation. New Connections: Increasing Diversity of RWJF Programming. 2009. http://www.rwjf-newconnections.org/. Accessed October 11, 2011.

58. Robert Wood Johnson Foundation. Summer Medical and Dental Education Program. 2012. http://www.smdep.org. Accessed June 3, 2012.

59. Harold Amos Medical Faculty Development Program. 2011. http://www.amfdp.org/. Accessed October 10, 2011.

3

Public Health Workforce and Education in the United States

Connie J. Evashwick

The public health workforce is a highly diverse collection of personnel representing multiple disciplines with a wide variety of career paths and employment settings, numerous types of formal and informal training, and a broad range of job functions. In the United States formal education in public health is offered by schools of public health, master's degree programs, clinical professionals' programs with specialties in public health, and colleges and universities. In addition, many of those working in public health come from other disciplines and have no formal training in public health. On-the-job training and continuing education for the workforce are provided by government public health departments, nonprofit organizations, medical centers and health systems, commercial educational enterprises, and various other organizations. This chapter presents an overview of the public health workforce and its education, emphasizing the heterogeneity and related complexities and outlining key considerations for shaping the public health workforce of the twenty-first century. For many of the relevant issues, however, the data required for precise analysis are lacking.

Background

The United States' Healthy People initiative recognizes the importance of public health manpower to the nation's health. One of the *Healthy People 2020* goals is "to ensure that Federal, State, Tribal, and local health agencies have the necessary infrastructure to effectively provide essential public health services." The report continues:

> Public health infrastructure is fundamental to the provision and execution of public health services at all levels. . . . Public health infrastructure includes 3 key components that enable public health organizations . . . to deliver public health services. These components are:
>> A capable and qualified workforce
>> Up-to-date data and information systems
>> Public health agencies capable of assessing and responding to public health needs.[1]

Similarly, the Institute of Medicine opened its 2003 report *Who Will Keep the Public Healthy?* as follows: "In a world where health threats range from AIDS and bioterrorism to an epidemic of obesity, the need for an effective public health system is as urgent as it has ever been. An effective public health system requires well-educated public health professionals" (p. 1).[2] Clearly, a workforce that is adequate in quantity and satisfactory in quality is essential to a well-functioning public health system.

The Affordable Care Act of 2010 (ACA) reinforces the importance of the workforce by including a lengthy list of provisions pertaining to the supply and training of health care, including public health professionals.[3] These provisions focus on direct training; infrastructure with education and training components; and workforce analysis, planning, and enumeration, among others. Elements of the ACA also reflect the public health workforce issues for which there is a consensus on national priorities for the coming years.

In summary, the public health workforce is one of the foundations of a healthy society. Despite its significance, counting and characterizing that workforce can be problematic.

Definition and Enumeration

The public health workforce in the United States can be described as a multidimensional mosaic of positions, functions, disciplines, degrees, and licenses. Enumerating and characterizing the public health workforce are elusive tasks. Job descriptions vary from setting to setting. Public health professionals come from an array of disciplines and formal education programs. Educational backgrounds vary widely, as do professional certifications. In an effort to capture this diversity, the Institute of Medicine defines a public health professional as follows: a person educated in public health or a related discipline who is employed to improve health through a population focus (p. 4).[2]

The most recent detailed, comprehensive enumeration of the U.S. public

health workforce was done in 2000 (see box).[4] The taxonomy of jobs consti-
tuting the public health workforce was based on categories used by the U.S.
Bureau of Labor Statistics, refined by the Bureau of Health Professions of the
Health Resources and Services Administration (HRSA). This list of occupa-
tions may be revised at a future date, but it offers a baseline. The study concluded that there were nearly 450,000 people working in public health jobs,
primarily for government agencies.[4] Of these, 34 percent worked at the local
level, 33 percent at the state level, and 19 percent at the federal level. About
14 percent worked outside of government settings, including those employed
by schools of public health, such as faculty, researchers, and managers. There
were 158 public health workers per 100,000 population, compared with 254
physicians and 778 nurses per 100,000 population.[5]

In the absence of comprehensive workforce data, one method of analyzing

Public Health (PH) Workforce by Title

Professional

Administrative
Alcohol and substance abuse counselor, including addiction counselor
Biostatistician
Clinical counselor
Environmental engineer
Environmental scientist and specialist
Epidemiologist
Health economist
Health educator
Health information system/computer specialist
Health services manager/health services administrator
Infection control/disease investigator
Licensure/inspection/regulatory specialist
Marriage and family therapist
Medical and public health and community social worker
Mental health counselor
Mental health/substance abuse social worker
Occupational safety and health specialist
PH attorney or hearing officer
PH dental worker
PH dentist
PH educator
PH laboratory scientist
PH nurse
PH nutritionist
PH optometrist

PH pharmacist
PH physical therapist
PH physician
PH policy analyst
PH program specialist
PH student
PH veterinarian/animal control specialist
Psychiatric nurse
Psychiatrist
Psychologist, mental health provider
Public relations/public information/health communications/media specialist
Substance abuse and behavioral disorders counselor
Other PH professional

Technical

Community outreach/field-worker
Computer specialist
Environmental engineering technician and technologist
Environmental science and protection technician
Health information systems/data analyst
Investigations specialist
Occupational safety and health technician and technologist
PH laboratory technician and technologist
Other paraprofessional
Other PH technician
Other protective service worker

Clerical/Support

Administrative business staff
Administrative support staff
Food services/housekeeping
Patient services
Other service/maintenance

Volunteers

Volunteer health administrator
Volunteer PH educator
Volunteer other paraprofessional

Source: Gebbie K, Standish GE, Merrill J. *The Public Health Work Force Enumeration 2000.* U.S. DHHS, Health Resources and Services Administration. HRSA/ATPM Cooperative Agreement No. U76 AH 00001-03. New York: Columbia University School of Nursing Center for Health Policy; December 2000. Based on CHP/CHPr+ classification scheme, modified by the Federal Standard Occupational Classification System, 1997.

the characteristics of the public health workforce is to examine each distinct public health profession. The professional associations representing each discipline often have relevant information and data. For example, nurses are the single most prevalent public health professional (setting aside clerical and administrative support staff), representing nearly 11 percent of the public health workforce. The American Public Health Association's Section on Nursing, the American Nurses Association, and the Quad Council of Public Health Nursing Organizations are sources of information about public health nurses. Epidemiologists are one of the most clearly defined public health professionals. The Council of State and Territorial Epidemiologists gathers information on careers, continuing education opportunities, and workforce issues pertaining to epidemiologists who work for public health departments. Public health laboratory specialists, health educators, and environmental health specialists are other sectors of the public health workforce that have specific professional associations that offer workforce data. Many of the best known national professional associations related to public health are listed in the appendix. Many states also have such professional associations.

Associations representing employment settings are another source of information about the public health workforce. The Association of State and Territorial Health Officials (ASTHO), the National Association of County and City Health Officials (NACCHO), and the National Association of Local Boards of Health all gather data on employees of their respective public health organizations. The National Association of Community Health Centers has select information about staff, services, funding, policy, and other topics related to public health infrastructure. Associations that represent public health workplace settings are also included in the appendix.

The global public health workforce is even more challenging to count and characterize. The World Health Organization (WHO) estimates the number of professionals and paraprofessionals working in health throughout the world. In many developing countries, the distinction between community and individual health blur. For example, the WHO uses a job classification system that includes physicians (urban and rural), nurses, midwives, environmental and public health workers, community and traditional workers, health workers, and health managers.[6] Counts are available by occupational title and by country, but no international statistics exist for comparison with U.S. studies. It suffices to know that many public health professionals educated or trained in the United States work abroad for all or part of their careers, and these individuals are not included in the U.S. public health workforce while they are employed outside the country.

Educating the Public Health Workforce

Unlike medicine, nursing, or other health professions, public health does not require education at any particular type of school that is directly linked to licensing or certification in the public health field. Hence, many of those holding both professional and nonprofessional positions in public health have no formal training in public health, or if they do, it was part of a course or component of education in another field. Formal academic training in public health is conducted by the nation's schools of public health, programs in public health, clinical disciplines that offer subspecialty training in public health, and, increasingly, universities and community colleges that offer undergraduate majors and minors in general public health or public health specialty fields. In addition, universities in other countries offer training in public health in a variety of formats. This section highlights major sources of formal training in public health in the United States.

As of 2012, there were forty-nine schools of public health in the United States accredited by the Council on Education for Public Health (CEPH), with nearly 8,000 graduates per year. The numbers of schools and graduates have been increasing steadily, as shown in figures 3.1 and 3.2, respectively. Over the past three decades, the number of graduates with master's degrees increased from 2,033 to 7,737 per year, and those earning doctoral degrees increased from 190 to 1,220. The total number of students enrolled in schools of public health in 2010 was over 26,000. Between 1974–1975 and 2010–2011, schools of public health conferred a total of 164,000 master's and doctoral degrees.[7]

Schools of public health offer more than sixteen distinct degrees and many more concentrations. The most common degrees are listed in table 3.1. Schools of public health are represented by the Association of Schools of Public Health (ASPH), which produces an annual data report (a list of current schools, degrees, and data on schools and students can be found at http://www.asph.org). Accreditation by CEPH is designed to ensure some degree of standardization and quality of the educational content.

Programs in public health typically grant the master's of public health (MPH) degree. As of 2011, there were eighty-three programs accredited by CEPH, mirroring the growth in the number of schools.[8] Approximately one in every five students enrolled in an accredited master's degree program in public health is in a CEPH-accredited program (more than 6,000 students in 2010). Information about CEPH-accredited MPH programs can be found through CEPH, the Association for Prevention Teaching and Research (APTR), and the Association of Accredited Public Health Programs (AAPHP). Specialty training at the master's level can also be obtained in epidemiology, environmental

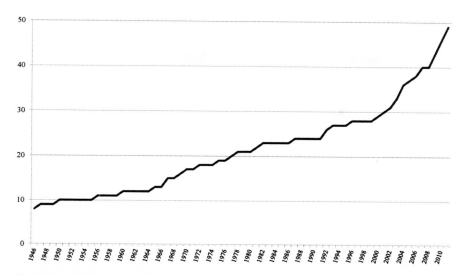

Figure 3.1. Number of schools of public health, 1946–2011. *Source:* Association of Schools of Public Health.

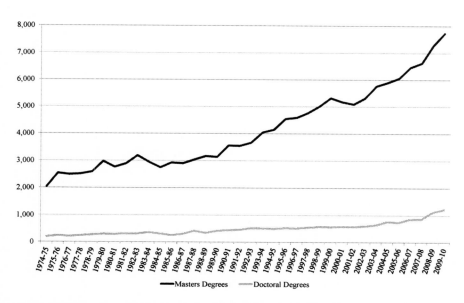

Figure 3.2. Number of master's and doctoral degrees awarded by schools of public health, 1974–1975 through 2009–2010. *Source:* Association of Schools of Public Health.

Table 3.1. Common Graduate Degrees Offered by Schools of Public Health*	
Acronym	**Degree**
Master's degrees	
MPH	Master of public health
MS	Master of science
MSPH	Master of science in public health
MHA	Master of health (hospital) administration
MHSA	Master of health service administration
Doctoral degrees	
DrPH	Doctor of public health
ScD	Doctor of science
PhD	Doctor of philosophy
Joint and dual degrees	
MPH/MD	Master of public health/doctor of medicine
MPH/JD	Master of public health/juris doctor
MPH/MSW	Master of public health/master of social work
MPH/MSN	Master of public health/master of nursing
MPH/MBA	Master of public health/master of business administration

* Other master's, doctoral, and dual degrees are offered, but they are less common and often indicate a specialty subject area.
Source: Association of Schools of Public Health Annual Data Report, 2010.

and occupational health, health administration, health education, and other related degrees. There are separate accreditation and professional associations for these discipline-specific fields (see the appendix).

Many programs that are not accredited by either CEPH or other accrediting bodies also offer training in public health, although the content is more variable than in accredited programs. The number of online universities offering graduate and undergraduate training in public health has grown over the past two decades, reflecting the general growth in online education. Reliable data on the total number of programs and graduates are not available. In 2011 one online source (http://www.gradschools.com/) listed 836 graduate schools and programs in public health, including 170 awarding certificates, 652 awarding master's degrees, and 233 awarding doctoral degrees.[9]

At the undergraduate level, public health has emerged as one of the fastest growing majors and areas of concentration. Undergraduate programs range from those offering specialty degrees such as environmental health, with education oriented toward specific career paths, to those offering general degrees in public health with broad liberal arts training. In 2011 the College Board listed 511 colleges with majors in public health, 29 of which were housed in CEPH-accredited schools of public health or CEPH-accredited programs.[10] In the coming decade, growth in public health education at the undergraduate level is expected to increase in both four-year universities and community colleges.

From the perspective of continuing education in public health, numerous public and private organizations offer training in a variety of formats accessible to those who cannot be full-time students. Private-public partnerships are common. For example, public health training centers are based largely in schools of public health and are funded by the HRSA to offer training to state and local health departments (http://www.phtc.org). This national network promotes the delivery of training that is relevant to local community needs while facilitating the sharing of these programs throughout the nation. Most schools of public health offer select continuing education programs, and many virtual universities offer online education pertinent to general public health or to specific topics. The National Public Health Leadership Development Institute and the Public Health Foundation are examples of two nonprofit organizations that offer training in public health. ASTHO and NACCHO provide continuing education targeted specifically at those working in and with government public health entities. The American Public Health Association draws 11,000 to 13,000 professionals for an extensive annual meeting covering a wide range of public health topics. Accrediting agencies, ranging from the Joint Commission on the Accreditation of Healthcare Organizations to the Public Health Accreditation Board, require documentation of training or currency for those working in positions directly or indirectly related to public health. These myriad educational and training opportunities reflect that there is no single requirement by governmental or private sources. Thus, the ongoing educational needs of the public health workforce are determined by each employer, discipline, or professional society.

Competency-based education

As a practice-oriented field, public health education emphasizes a pragmatic approach to training, based on the defined competencies needed to work in the field. ASPH has been a driving force in developing competency sets as the foundation for graduate education in CEPH-accredited schools and programs (for details on educational competencies for different levels and aspects of public health education, go to http://www.asph.org/competencies). Core competencies for the MPH degree include epidemiology, biostatistics, social and behavioral science, environmental science, and health management and policy. Cross-cutting competencies include professionalism, leadership, systems thinking, communications and informatics, diversity and culture, program planning, and public health biology. In addition to devising content for those specializing in public health, ASPH has worked with the Association of American Colleges and Universities to develop a statement of learning outcomes for undergraduates (http://www.asph.org/competencies/Learning Outcomes). This construct is based on the "educated citizen" concept expressed by the Institute of Medicine, with the goal that everyone attending a college or university has a basic understanding of public health principles that they can apply to their individual behavior and role in society.

The Council on Linkages between Academia and Public Health Practice and other professional associations have also contributed extensively to articulating the competencies required for the optimal performance of the public health workforce. The Council on Linkages revised its competencies in 2010; they are aimed at those actively working in the field of public health and distinguish among entry-level, midlevel, and senior-level practitioners (http://www.phf.org). *Core Competencies for Interprofessional Collaborative Practice,* released in 2011, was developed jointly by ASPH and the national associations of five clinical disciplines—medicine, nursing, pharmacy, dentistry, and osteopathy.[11] These competencies reflect the recognition that health professionals of all disciplines need to work together, taking a team approach to the care of individuals as well as communities. Specialty competencies may apply to particular tasks or functions within public health, such as emergency preparedness, global health, or public health informatics.

National licensure and certification

There is no licensure for public health professionals per se. Those entering specific disciplines, such as nursing, take the appropriate licensing examination for their discipline and state. A general license may or may not have any components related to public health. For example, a nurse working in a public health department would take the state licensing examination for registered nurses; there is no separate examination for nurses working in public health clinics. A clinical health professional might supplement a general license with a subspecialty certification pertinent to public health. For example, physicians specializing in environmental and occupational health would first graduate from an accredited medical school, sit for the licensing examination in their state, and then choose to pursue a specialty in occupational medicine, awarded by a national specialty board within the discipline of medicine.

Public health is perhaps one of the last health professions to add individual certification as a measure of professional qualification. The National Board of Public Health Examiners began offering an examination in 2008 that awards the Certified in Public Health (CPH) designation upon successful completion. To be eligible, a person must have an MPH or equivalent degree from a CEPH-accredited school or program. Licensing or clinical education is not a prerequisite to obtaining the CPH credential; however, CPH renewal requires continuing education.

Workforce Issues for the Twenty-First Century

The WHO has laid out the structural components pertinent to having a strong health system.[12] These include adequate numbers of workers with appropriate competencies, functional support systems, and an enabling environment. The U.S. public health workforce has been examined over the past half century by the Institute of Medicine, the federal government, and a variety of other public and private institutions. The challenges to achieving the goals of a well-trained workforce of adequate size and appropriate expertise and conducive work settings have been relatively persistent over the past decade. They have become even more prominent due to recent trends in health care, public health, education, the economy, and social demographics.

Shortages

The U.S. public health system faces a severe shortage in the number of workers available due to retirement and problems related to retention and recruitment. Retirement of the baby boom generation is one factor. Public health, like other health professions, will see the retirement of an estimated 20 percent or more of the total workforce by 2020. An analysis by ASPH in 2007–2008 estimated a shortfall of as many as 250,000 master's-level public health practitioners by 2020, with up to 100,000 government public health employees eligible to retire as of 2012.[13] This retirement trend will not only reduce the number of people working in public health but also substantially change the mix of senior managers with experience and more junior staff with less experience but perhaps a greater propensity for the use of technology. Hence, the change in the composition of the workforce may result in changes in operations and practices.

In addition, the economic downturn in the United States between 2008 and 2011 affected many state and local public health departments. NACCHO reported that more than half the local health departments throughout the nation experienced job losses between 2008 and 2010, with a total of 29,000 jobs cut.[14] Similarly, ASTHO reported that 89 percent of state health agencies experienced workforce reductions from 2008 through early 2011, with a total of 14,700 lost jobs.[15] Although these functions might be taken over by other workers or accomplished by work redesign in the short term, the dramatic decrease in the public health workforce means fewer workers available to meet the increased demands placed on the public health system by the ACA of 2010 and other recent environmental trends.

Recruiting workers into the field of public health is also challenging. Public health is poorly understood as a field, let alone a career. Initiatives such as the "This Is Public Health" campaign and fellowship programs run by the Centers for Disease Control and Prevention (CDC) strive to recruit young people into the field early in their educational careers. A sobering fact is that while many students are incurring increasingly large financial debts in pursuit of a formal education,[16] salaries in many facets of public health, particularly government and nonprofit positions, are less than those paid for comparable positions in other fields or other careers in health care.

Alignment of needs and skills

The Global Independent Commission on Education of Health Professionals for the 21st Century advocates a systems approach, starting with a determination of what functions need to be performed to address the problems of the health care delivery system and then shaping professional education accordingly.[17] As noted earlier, the current approach to training the public health workforce is a combination of no training, discipline-specific clinical training with public health as an add-on, and topic-specific continuing education responding to the latest crisis or trend. Only a relatively small percentage of the public health workforce has any core training specifically related to public health.

Ideally, the goal is to match the needs of the health system with the skills of those who are trained to work in it. Education for public health has become competency driven, which raises several questions: Which competencies apply? To which workers? For what purposes? If workers can demonstrate "competence," does this have a direct impact on the health of the public or the performance of the public health system? As workers retire or change positions, what are the implications for continuing education? How does education of the workforce relate to the public health needs of the community?

The multiple sets of competencies pertinent to health professionals complicate the responses to these questions. A 2011 cataloging of such competencies found no fewer than fifteen sets of them, including those for clinicians of various disciplines, health care administrators and policy analysts, ethicists, emergency responders, environmental health specialists, and health educators, among others.[18] In addition, there are competencies for formal university programs and other competencies for those already employed in a public health setting.

The importance of lifelong continuing education is also apparent. As the older generation of workers retires, their replacements or those advancing to new positions may need different job skills. As the public health environment changes due to technology, globalization, advances in science, or the emergence of new diseases, updated knowledge and commensurate skills will be necessary, even if personnel have a solid foundation of basic competencies.

New perspectives continue to inform education and expectations about workers' knowledge and skills. A trend toward systems thinking and the nonstop advancement of a broad range of technologies warrant a consideration of how educational competencies relate to future job needs. For example, in the twenty years between 1990 and 2010, computer technology and the science of informatics completely changed how surveillance—one of the core public health functions—is conducted. Mapping of the outbreak and spread of disease has changed dramatically: Whereas physicians were once required to report individual patients with contagious diseases, now highly sophisticated geographic information systems track outbreaks in multiple dimensions. In the past, communication involved telephone calls from laboratories to public health experts, but today, social media alerts reach hundreds of laypeople instantaneously, and, conversely, hundreds of laypeople alert national media and health agencies with frontline information during emergencies. Preparing the public health workforce to manage such drastic changes and to employ emerging technology requires ongoing education and personnel change management.

Interprofessional collaboration

Collaboration among professionals from different disciplines has been touted by past generations and periodically experiences a revival in popularity; then it wanes as the practical challenges of implementation set in. Since 2010, interprofessional collaboration has once again come to the forefront.[11] Recognition of the multiple factors that affect disease prevention, chronic disease management, and health promotion has combined with ACA-related changes in the health care delivery system to emphasize that the creation of healthy communities and healthy individuals cannot be achieved by individuals acting alone. Public health professionals have typically taken a broad perspective, and now seems to be an appropriate time to take an interdisciplinary approach to prevention and population health.

Global health

The globalization of the world's economies has led to the realization that no country can stand alone. Public health calamities such as SARS, avian flu, and the ongoing challenges of HIV/AIDS have reinforced the notion that "public health is global health."[19] Immigration continues to expand the diversity of the U.S. population.[20] All these forces mean that the public health workforce must be cognizant of the impact of global health on day-to-day tasks, whether in the Badlands of South Dakota or on the beaches of Florida.

The Global Independent Commission on Education of Health Professionals for the 21st Century emphasizes the need for a global perspective when it comes to educating and deploying public health professionals.[17] Universities and public health institutions across the country have not yet responded to this challenge, but their programs are likely to evolve as it becomes increasingly clear how a diverse environment affects the daily tasks of all public health workers—from the receptionist who needs to be multilingual to the physician who needs to promote vaccinations within the context of a recent immigrant's culture.

A few schools of public health have established specific training programs in global health. Others have taken the approach of globalizing the entire curriculum—that is, infusing global awareness and global relevancy into all courses and all degree programs. These are still in the minority, however. A set of global health competencies was recently developed by more than 380 health care practitioners from around the world, both in academia and in practice. These competencies include the main domains or content areas in which public health practitioners specializing in global health should be proficient, including capacity strengthening, collaboration and partnering, ethical and professional practice, health equity and social justice, program management, sociocultural and political awareness, and strategic analysis.

Cultural competence and health literacy

One of the most common manifestations of globalization is the need for cultural sensitivity and cultural competence. For example, in one large county in California, residents spoke 109 languages, and the county printed all materials in the 18 most common languages. Public health practitioners who are trying to influence behaviors must be aware of their constituents' social and behavioral foundations if they are going to be successful in promoting change. National standards on culturally and linguistically appropriate services (CLAS) are frequently used as a reference point for health care practitioners.[21] The CLAS standards are targeted at health care organizations, but they can also be used to make individual clinical practices more culturally and linguistically accessible. The fourteen standards are organized around three main themes: culturally competent care (standards 1–3), language access services (standards 4–7), and organizational supports for cultural competence (standards 8–14). According to the U.S. Department of Health and Human Services (DHHS) Office of Minority Health, "The principles and activities of culturally and linguistically appropriate services should be integrated throughout an organization and undertaken in partnership with the communities being served."[21] By inference, public health professionals must be knowledgeable about cultural competence in order to implement this mandate.

The current focus on health literacy is yet another manifestation of the need to create messages that can be understood and acted on by individuals, families, and communities. Health literacy is defined as the degree to which individuals have the capacity to obtain, process, and understand the basic health information needed to make appropriate health decisions and utilize the services required to prevent or treat illness. The HRSA and CDC have both acknowledged the importance of health literacy to health care and public health professionals and have created tools to promote health literacy.[22, 23]

Teaching technologies and innovations

Scientific knowledge, biomedical and communications technologies, and innovations of all types have drastically changed public health from milk wagons delivering supplies for newborns to highly sophisticated jobs employing advanced technology to facilitate access and learning. Public health informatics has evolved as its own field of specialization, with competencies and support from professional associations.[24] Geographic information systems are now widely utilized to conduct disease surveillance and have been incorporated into classroom education. Distance learning and online educational options are so prevalent that there are more students enrolled online on any given day than sitting in classrooms. In brief, as the work of public health is increasingly facilitated by technology, those pursuing careers in public health—whether new students earning their first degrees or workforce veterans continuing their education—are enmeshed in technology as an integral part of their daily jobs. Similarly, educational institutions are evolving to offer education maximized by technology.

A strong, well-trained workforce is vital if a nation is to have a stellar public health system. Numerous challenges must be overcome to achieve this goal. Currently, the public health workforce in the United States is like a brightly colored Rubik's cube that can be organized and viewed from different perspectives for different purposes. The tasks of identifying, enumerating, and characterizing the full workforce have yet to be accomplished, despite repeated attempts to do so. The issues that impact the workforce are many and can be dealt with most effectively if policies and programs are based on data and a consensus about future demand and supply.

The ACA of 2010 includes a number of provisions pertaining to the public health workforce. Some are aimed directly at resolving the issues mentioned here. Others are designed to implement the act's provisions to increase access to care but also have considerable implications for the public health workforce. Funding for many elements of the ACA was not forthcoming in 2011 or 2012 due to the nation's budget deficit. Which provisions are eventually funded and implemented over the first several years of the ACA's rollout will affect how and to what degree each of the above issues is addressed at the national level. In the meantime, local governments, nonprofit organizations, and for-profit companies must all work together to ensure a public health workforce that is adequate in size, appropriately trained, and motivated by a positive working environment.

Appendix: Entities Representing Public Health Disciplines or Functions

Association	Description	Website
American Association of Colleges of Nursing (AACN)	Baccalaureate and higher-degree nursing education programs	http://www.aacn.nche.edu/
American College of Preventive Medicine (ACPM)	2,600 physician members committed to disease prevention and health promotion	http://www.acpm.org/
American Medical Association (AMA)	Physicians, resident physicians, and medical students	http://www.ama-assn.org/
American Nurses Association (ANA)	3.1 million registered nurses	http://nursingworld.org/
American Public Health Association (APHA)	More than 30,000 individual public health professionals and 20,000 additional state and local affiliate members	http://www.apha.org/
Association for Prevention Teaching and Research (APTR)	Members represent the academic prevention community	http://www.aptrweb.org/
Association of Academic Health Centers (AAHC)	More than 100 academic health centers nationwide	http://www.aahcdc.org/
Association of Accredited Public Health Programs (AAPHP)	21 CEPH-accredited public health programs	http://www.mphprograms.org/
Association of American Medical Colleges (AAMC)	134 accredited U.S. and 17 accredited Canadian medical schools; approximately 400 major teaching hospitals and health systems	https://www.aamc.org/
Association of Public Health Laboratories (APHL)	53 state and 41 local governmental public health labs	http://www.aphl.org/
Association of Schools of Public Health (ASPH)	49 CEPH-accredited graduate schools of public health	http://www.asph.org
Association of State and Territorial Health Officials (ASTHO)	59 state and territorial health officials	http://www.astho.org
Association of University Programs in Health Administration (AUPHA)	180 graduate and undergraduate university programs in North America (U.S. and Canada)	http://www.aupha.org

Appendix: Entities Representing Public Health Disciplines or Functions, continued

Association	Description	Website
Centers for Disease Control and Prevention (CDC)	Major component of the Department of Health and Human Services that is the national leader in developing and applying disease prevention and control, environmental health, health promotion, and health education activities to improve the health of the U. S. population	http://www.cdc.gov
Council of State and Territorial Epidemiologists (CSTE)	Members are state and territorial public health epidemiologists	http://cste.org
Health Resources and Services Administration (HRSA)	Agency of the Department of Health and Human Services responsible for improving access to health care services for people who are uninsured, isolated, or medically vulnerable	http://www.hrsa.gov
National Association of Community Health Centers (NACHC)	More than 1,200 health centers and 8,000 delivery sites	www.nachc.com
National Association of County and City Health Officials (NACCHO)	1,450 local health departments (comprising more than 13,000 health officials and their staffs)	http://www.naccho.org
National Association of Local Boards of Health (NALBOH)	Boards of local health departments	http://www.nalboh.org
National Board of Public Health Examiners (NBPHE)	Certifies public health professionals with the CPH credential (which requires a master's degree from an accredited school of public health or program)	http://www.nbphe.org
National Environmental Health Association (NEHA)	4,500+ environmental health professionals in the public and private sectors, academia, and the uniformed services; a majority are employed by state and county health departments	http://www.neha.org

Appendix: Entities Representing Public Health Disciplines or Functions, continued		
Association	**Description**	**Website**
National Network of Public Health Institutes (NNPHI)	National membership network committed to helping public health institutes promote and sustain improved health and wellness for all	http://www.nnphi.org
National Public Health Leadership Development Network	Consortium of organizations and individuals from academic institutions; national and international organizations; and local, state, and federal agencies dedicated to advancing the practice of public health leadership	http://www.heartlandcenters.slu.edu/nln/index.html
Quad Council of Public Health Nursing Organizations	Current member organizations are the Association of State and Territorial Directors of Nursing (ASTDN), the ANA's Council on Nursing Practice and Economics, the Association of Community Health Nursing Educators (ACHNE), and the APHA's Section of Public Health Nursing	http://www.achne.org/i4a/pages/index.cfm?pageid=3292
Society for Public Health Education (SOPHE)	Health education professionals and students	http://www.sophe.org
World Health Organization (WHO)	Collects data on countries throughout the world, including health and health workforce statistics	http://www.who.org

Source: Compiled by the Association of Schools of Public Health, 2011. Current as of July 2011; information may change without notice.

Notes

The author would like to acknowledge the contributions of Kristin Dolinski, Elizabeth Weist, Jamie DiGiacomo, John McElligott, and Harrison Spencer, MD, MPH.

1. U.S. DHHS, Centers for Disease Control and Prevention. *Healthy People 2020.* http://www.cdc.gov/healthypeople2020. Accessed July 25, 2011.

2. Gebbie K, Rosenstock L, Hernandez L, eds. *Who Will Keep the Public Healthy? Educating Public Health Professionals for the 21st Century.* Washington, DC: National Academies Press; 2003.

3. American Public Health Association. *The Affordable Care Act's Public Health Workforce Provisions: Opportunities and Challenges*. Center for Public Health Policy issue brief. Washington, DC: American Public Health Association; June 2011.

4. Gebbie K, Standish GE, Merrill J. *The Public Health Work Force Enumeration 2000*. U.S. DHHS, Health Resources and Services Administration. HRSA/ATPM Cooperative Agreement No. U76 AH 00001-03. New York: Columbia University School of Nursing Center for Health Policy; December 2000.

5. U.S. DHHS. Health U.S., 2007. http://www.cdc.gov/nchs/data/hus/hus07.pdf. Accessed July 28, 2011.

6. World Health Organization. http://www.who.org. Accessed July 25, 2011.

7. Association of Schools of Public Health. Member schools: Special data analysis. http://www.ASPH.org/document.cfm?page=200. Accessed July 29, 2011.

8. Council on Education for Public Health. http://www.ceph.org. Accessed August 14, 2011.

9. Mintz J. The changing landscape of public health education. Paper presented at the Association of Schools of Public Health Deans' Retreat, July 22, 2011, Montreal Canada.

10. College Board. http://www.collegeboard.org. Accessed July 12, 2011.

11. Interprofessional Education Collaborative Expert Panel. *Core Competencies for Interprofessional Collaborative Practice: Report of an Expert Panel*. Washington, DC: Interprofessional Education Collaborative; 2011. https://www.aamc.org/download/186750/data/core_competencies.pdf. Accessed August 9, 2011.

12. World Health Organization. *Towards Better Leadership and Management in Health*. Working Paper No. 10. Geneva: WHO Press, 2007. http://www.WHO/HSS/healthsystems/2007.3. Accessed August 14, 2011.

13. Association of Schools of Public Health. *Confronting the Public Health Workforce Crisis*. ASPH policy brief. Washington, DC: ASPH; December 2008.

14. National Association of County and City Health Officials. *Local Health Department Job Losses and Program Cuts: Findings from January 2011 Survey and 2010 National Profile Study*. Washington, DC: NACCHO; 2011. http://www.NACCHO.org/jobloss. Accessed August 14, 2011.

15. Association of State and Territorial Health Officials. *Budget Cuts Continue to Affect the Health of Americans: Update*. Research brief. Arlington, VA: ASTHO; May 2011.

16. U.S. Department of Education, National Center for Education Statistics. *1995–96, 1999–2000, 2003–04, and 2007–08 National Postsecondary Student Aid Study*. Web table 3. Washington, DC: U.S. Department of Education; September 2010. http://www.nces.ed.gov/pubsearch/pubsinfo.asp?pubid=2010180. Accessed July 6, 2011.

17. Frenk J, Chen L, et al. Health professionals for a new century: Transforming education to strengthen health systems in an interdependent world. *Lancet*. 2010;376:1234–1258.

18. Association of Schools of Public Health. Internal analysis of competency sets. June 2011.

19. Friend L, Bentley M, Buekens P, Burke D, Frenk J, Klag M, Spencer H. Global health is public health. *Lancet*. 2010;375:536–537.

20. Hobb, F, Stoops N. *Demographic Trends in the 20th Century*. U.S. Bureau of the Census, CENSR-4. Washington, DC: U.S. Department of Commerce; November 2002:71–114. http://www.census.gov/publications. Accessed August 11, 2011.

21. U.S. DHHS, Office of Minority Health. National Standards on Culturally and Linguistically Appropriate Services. http://www.minorityhealth.hhs.gov/templates/browse.aspx?lvl=2&lvlid=15. Accessed August 11, 2011.

22. U.S. DHHS, Health Resources and Services Administration. About Health Literacy. http://www.hrsa.gov/publichealth/healthliteracy/healthlitabout.html. Accessed August 11, 2011.

23. U.S. DHHS, Centers for Disease Control and Prevention. CDC Health Literacy for Public Health Professionals, On-Line Training. http://www.cdc.gov/healthcommunication/. Accessed August 11, 2011.

24. U.S. DHHS, Centers for Disease Control and Prevention. Competencies for Public Health Informaticians, 2009. http://www.cdc.gov/InformaticsCompetencies/. Accessed August 14, 2011.

4

The Role of Community-Oriented Primary Care in Improving Health Care

Samuel C. Matheny

Over the last few decades, there has been a growing interest in the relationship of primary care to the health of communities. Several factors have contributed to this movement. First, there is increasing awareness that although the United States spends a greater proportion of its national budget on health care than any other country, Americans' health lags significantly behind that of residents of other developed countries in many areas. Second, there is new and convincing evidence that the presence of a robust primary care system is strongly connected to positive health outcomes. This is complicated by a third factor—that is, the significant shortage of primary care providers in the country. This factor may challenge the successful adaptation to changes in the organization and financing of health care. Last, there has been an increased emphasis on community participation in decision making, which has also influenced health care delivery. It is important to examine the principles of primary care and community health more completely to understand how they are interactive and mutually dependent. Addressing the health care of a community along with the care of individual patients is an essential function of the community-oriented primary care (COPC) concept.

Three of the individuals who had key roles in the leadership and development of both primary care and community health were William Willard, Nicholas Pisacano, and Kurt Deuschle. Willard, the founding dean of the University of Kentucky College of Medicine, was the chief author of a report from the American Medical Association entitled *Meeting the Challenge of Family Practice*.[1] The Willard report, along with the Millis report (published the same year),[2] was a major incentive for the creation of a new primary care discipline called family practice. Pisacano, a professor of general practice at the same college, was one of the first individuals to consider the academic training needs for this new discipline and was responsible for the foundation of the American Board of Family Practice, now the American Board of Family Medicine. In 1960 Willard selected Deuschle to head the first Department of Community Medicine in the United States. The integration of these two movements—primary care and community medicine—began a decade later when the educational principles of family practice were solidified, and training programs in family practice and other primary care disciplines embraced many of the concepts of community medicine.

Defining Primary Care

The term *primary care* has been used for many years, but its current meaning was established in the middle of the twentieth century, most notably in the Millis report,[2] which led to the creation of the discipline of family practice. The definition was updated in 1996 by an Institute of Medicine (IOM) report, which stated: "Primary care is the provision of *integrated, accessible health care services* by clinicians who are *accountable* for addressing a large *majority of personal health care needs,* developing a *sustained partnership* with *patients,* and practicing in the *context of family and community.*"[3] This expanded the IOM's original 1978 definition of primary care to include the following concepts: (1) the inclusion of the patient and the family, (2) the role of the community, and (3) the integrated health care system, which the IOM thought would be an influential factor in health care delivery in the future (figure 4.1).

The IOM identified five categories to describe primary care : (1) the care provided by certain individuals, such as family physicians, general internists, pediatricians, physicians' assistants, and nurse practitioners; (2) a set of activities whose functions determine the boundaries of primary care; (3) an entry point in the system, which focuses on the first provider of care but includes care in hospitals or other settings defined as secondary or tertiary care; (4) a set of attributes as outlined in the 1978 definition, including care that is accessible, comprehensive, coordinated, continuous, and accountable; or (5) a strategy for organizing the health care system that includes the principles of COPC (reviewed later). In a statement issued prior to the IOM report, the chair of the Committee on the Future of Primary Care commented: "Exemplary primary care requires an understanding of the community, defined by the committee as the population served, whether patients or not. This implies an understanding

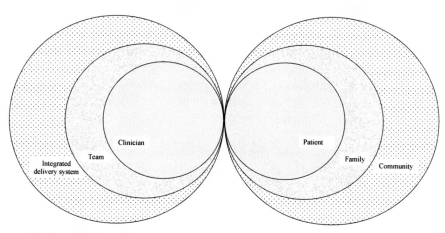

Figure 4.1. Interdependence of the constituents of primary care, showing the centrality of the patient-clinician relationship in the context of family and community, furthered by teams and integrated delivery systems. *Source:* National Research Council. *Primary Care: America's Health in a New Era.* Washington, DC: National Academies Press; 1996.

of what is happening in the community, knowledge of the major causes of morbidity and mortality in the population served, and a strengthened link between primary care and population-based public health services."[4] The authors of the report believed that although clarifying the definition would be advantageous to policy makers, the complexity of the issues surrounding primary care demands a multidimensional approach to policy decisions.

Relation of Primary Care to Health Outcomes and Cost

In recent years, it has become apparent that well-organized primary care can improve health outcomes and reduce costs. The proof for these conclusions is robust, but it depends somewhat on the definition of primary care. Studies evaluating the efficacy of primary care have centered around three definitions: (1) the specialty of primary care physicians, such as general pediatrics and family medicine; (2) the functions of primary care, including being the usual source of care and having responsibility for first contact, continuity, comprehensiveness, and coordination of services; and (3) the system orientation of care, which involves the aggregation of primary care providers or ratio of primary care providers to specialists. The evidence appears to be the strongest in support of the second and third definitions of primary care.[5] In particular, in aggregate studies of states, the supply of primary care physicians was directly related to decreased overall mortality, especially infant mortality, even when controlling for income levels and many other variables. This same effect has been demonstrated at the county level in the United States: all-cause mortality and mortality from two of the most common causes of death, heart disease and cancer, were lower when there were greater numbers of primary care physicians. These results were particularly significant in nonurban areas of the country.[6]

Studies have explored the impact on patients who have primary care physicians as their usual source of health care. It has been demonstrated that patients with primary care physicians have lower five-year mortality rates after controlling for other variables.[7] This finding has been corroborated when examining the impact of care provided by the nation's federally funded community health centers, which require the provision of primary care. These patients were more likely to have received preventive services than were patients in rural areas who obtained care from other sources; they were also more likely to have positive outcomes of pregnancy, with fewer low-birth-weight babies.[8]

The impact of primary care on preventive services is particularly noteworthy. Patients who received primary care had higher rates of immunization, screening, and health counseling. Other studies have demonstrated a positive effect on the delivery of care to adolescents, manifested by a decreased use of emergency rooms.[9] In the aggregate, states with better ratios of primary care physicians to population report more successful preventive activities, as evidenced by lower smoking rates and less obesity, among other measures.[10, 11]

A number of studies have explored the relationship between the costs of care and the availability of primary care services. They indicate that costs are significantly lower in areas with more primary care physicians per population. The same was true in studies of the impact of primary care on Medicare spending in the United States. These conclusions have been verified in a number of international studies—that is, countries with weaker primary care systems have significantly higher total health care costs.

In summary, there is good evidence that primary care has a strong positive influence on improving health and reducing costs.

Community Medicine and Community-Oriented Primary Care

Although the components of what would become known as community medicine have existed in the United States since the turn of the twentieth century, academic community medicine originated in 1960 when, as noted earlier, Deuschle became the nation's first chair of community medicine. His prior experience included a community health demonstration project between Cornell University and the U.S. Public Health Service on the Navajo reservation in the early 1950s, where medical students studied public health. He soon realized that students much preferred identifying community health problems in real-world settings than listening to theoretical discussions in a classroom.

Deuschle initially debated what to name the University of Kentucky's new department dealing with population health.[12] The goal was to develop an academic discipline around the study of specific populations and the delivery of health care, and he considered several options, such as *social medicine* and *population medicine*, but eventually decided on *community medicine* and defined the discipline as follows:

> Community medicine is the academic discipline that deals with the identification and solution of the health problems of communities or human population groups. This discipline, like internal medicine or pediatrics, has for its goal the solution of people's health problems through clinical application of the basic science disciplines of pathology, microbiology, behavioral sciences and biostatistics. However, community medicine considers people in groups or communities as well as individually, encompassing the traditional and relevant skills and knowledge of public health and preventive medicine along with the growing concern for the delivery of medical care. The epidemiologic method and body of knowledge are in a special position, linking the basic science portion of the discipline with the applied phase in the community.[13]

Required clerkships were organized in the fourth year of medical school, and they served as the prototype for several important concepts that were later adopted by other departments and clinical disciplines—family medicine in particular. The students' clerkships took place in assigned communities and were frequently multidisciplinary; students were expected to both assess the community by a formal process of a community diagnosis and perform an original epidemiologic project during the clerkship period. Community-based clinical clerkship rotations are now universal.

In the last fifty years, many schools of medicine have created departments of community medicine, most frequently as a joint title with another discipline. The terminology and content as they relate to scientific inquiry and clinical discipline vary considerably. A typology of community medicine methodologies has been described (table 4.1).[14] These different methodologies have been categorized as gradations of involvement, with the expanded

Table 4.1. Typology of Community Medicine Methodologies: Criteria

Methodology	Population of Interest	Health Assessment	Outcome	Community Involvement
Expanded primary care/quality improvement projects	Clinic patients	Individual patient	Improved screening or treatment	No
Community-oriented primary care	Population covered by clinic	Clinic population	Project outcome	Variable
Community-based health/participatory research	Specific population	Community/population	Community involvement and improvement	Yes, significant
Public health	City, state, country	By state, county, etc.	Reduce risk factors	Government only

Source: Gavagan T. A systematic review of COPC: Evidence for effectiveness. *J Health Care Poor Underserved.* 2008;19(3):965.

primary care model as the most modest level and the traditional community-based health and public health strategies requiring the greatest resources and involvement.

One community medicine methodology had its beginnings in South Africa in 1940, when two young physicians, Sidney and Emily Kark, founded the Pholela Health Centre. This unit, which was the model for a network of similar units around the country, was set up to function independently of any existing governmental health service and was tasked to provide comprehensive health services by "combin[ing] curative and preventive services, including . . . the prevention and treatment of disease . . . health education . . . local cooperation and community responsibility."[15] Local community health workers were involved in the center, and two innovations in health care were implemented. One was to create an initial defined area (IDA) for intensive study and service, and the second was to develop a household health census. After a short time, patients in the IDA demonstrated significant health improvements, and subsequent activities evolved into specific interventions aimed at changing the health-related behaviors of individuals and families, quantifying outcomes to determine which interventions should be prioritized, and designing evaluation methodologies. These activities demanded improved systems for the collection of data, such as demographic information on the population, special information on determinants of health, and health and morbidity data. The concept of the initial clinic expanded, and it became an important site for the education of medical students. The Karks moved to Israel, where they continued their work and were responsible for training many clinicians from around the world, including the United States.

The Karks' model became known as community-oriented primary care and was defined as "a continuous process by which primary health care is provided to a defined population on the basis of its defined health needs by the planned integration of public health with primary care practice."[16] Five cardinal questions formed the basis for COPC:

1. What is the community's state of health?
2. What are the factors responsible for this health state?
3. What is being done about it?
4. What more can be done, and what is the expected outcome?
5. What measures are needed to continue health surveillance of the community and to evaluate the effects of existing programs?

These questions led to the concept of the COPC cycle (figure 4.2).[17] Programs at George Washington University added another element—defining the community.

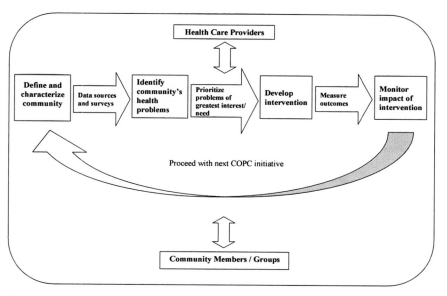

Figure 4.2. Community-oriented primary care cycle. *Source:* Emmanuel D. Jadhav. Used by permission.

Community-Oriented Primary Care Cycle

Defining the community

This preliminary step entails deciding on the geographic boundaries of the area to be studied.[18] The community may be based on a geographic, social, or economic distinction, or it may even comprise the members of a clinical practice, although Deuschle has argued that this is a "constituency," not a community.[19] The target population should be quantified by whatever information is accessible, which may be difficult. This information may be available from the practice itself, if it has a good system of data recovery, such as age or sex registers or computerized health records, or it may be necessary to extrapolate data from larger data sets, such as census data or school registers, in an attempt to estimate the incidence and prevalence rates of various conditions in the target area. In some cases, community surveys may be conducted. In addition, qualitative information about community resources may be obtained from focus groups or selected community informants.

Community characterization (community diagnosis)

These qualitative and quantitative data are compiled to determine which elements should be considered for prioritization (the next step). It has been pointed out that qualitative data are equally important as quantitative data in this process. The community diagnosis can be broad in scope, but as Abramson points out, this may make the task more difficult, and in most cases, the focus should be narrow to facilitate the potential for intervention.[20] For example, if both quantitative and qualitative data indicate that a community has a high rate of smoking, a number of related questions would be of interest: What is the prevalence of smoking in specific populations, such as teenagers or pregnant women? What is the documented relationship between smoking and other diseases in the community, such as cardiovascular disease or lung cancer? What are the community's attitudes about or understanding of smoking as a health problem? The community diagnosis may also include the status of health resources in a community, such as the adequacy of mental health facilities or long-term care facilities for the elderly.

Prioritization

The process of COPC usually involves prioritizing one intervention at a time, although that is not always the case. Community participation in this step is important. As previously mentioned, most clinicians need to determine which community problems to address first to avoid overwhelming the practice and limiting the potential for success.

Detailed problem assessment

There may be many potential options for intervention in a designated health problem, and all the various pieces of information need to be assimilated to ascertain what those options are before deciding on an action and planning an intervention. Some issues to consider may be the community's concern about the problem, the potential for effecting change, resources needed for the intervention, and the potential for health improvement.

Intervention and implementation

The intervention depends on the proven efficacy of the activity and the available resources. The Institute of Medicine has identified four levels of performance with respect to initiatives undertaken. The lowest grade of performance was assigned to interventions undertaken in response to a national initiative; the highest grade was identified in those that were specific to a community's identified health care needs.[21]

Evaluation

Evaluation of the selected intervention is most important for measuring effectiveness and planning future activities. Appropriate evaluation can provide positive reinforcement to health care workers and the community and can give them the incentive to continue their activities. Evaluation can focus on one aspect of the intervention or on the practice in general, measuring patient or community satisfaction, quality outcomes, clinical performance, cost-effectiveness, or service utilization.

In summary, the structure of COPC consists of a well-delineated cycle of decision components that form a continuous process. Community involvement is essential in most of these steps (particularly prioritization, assessment, intervention, and evaluation). There are several presumptions about the process, including the formation of teams to provide leadership. There is also some agreement that although many problems may be identified, these should be addressed sequentially rather than simultaneously. In this manner, a systematic approach has been designed for prioritizing and addressing the needs of a specific population through the provision of primary health care.[22]

Community-Oriented Primary Care around the World

It has now been more than seventy years since the COPC concept was first introduced, and it has become a major component of the primary care delivery system in a number of countries. Attempts have been made to introduce COPC into even more countries, led by the Hebrew University–Hadassah School of Public Health and Community Medicine in Jerusalem, Israel. In the last twenty years, the concept of COPC has been revived in the United Kingdom, with some degree of success, aided by pilot projects such as those initiated by the King's Fund. A new emphasis on increased responsibility for preventive medicine and the need to address the social determinants of health holds promise for the future success of health promotion and prevention.[17]

In Cuba, COPC is part of the training of family physicians working in health care teams of 600 to 800 people, and the principles of COPC have led to close working relationships with public health officials.[23] In Spain, there is a strong focus on primary care through the institution of family medicine programs. The COPC model has been developed throughout Catalonia, where it is now part of thirty primary care centers and the practices of more than 2,000 physicians in the area.[24]

In the United States, the COPC concept has found strong support in the Indian Health Service and in the Public Health Service's community health center program. Since the creation of the first community health center in Mound Bayou, Mississippi, the aim has been to develop community organizations to work with these centers, with the goal of increasing awareness of communities' problems through epidemiology, health education, and environmental programs and to link these initiatives to the primary care delivery system.[25] To a lesser extent, hospitals have also utilized the principles of COPC in community outreach programs. The Parkland Hospital system in Dallas, Texas, adopted a form of COPC to provide preventive and primary care in an integrated format, and it has promoted this model in spite of financial crises and budget cuts.[26]

Medical Education and Community-Oriented Primary Care

In the United States, the principles of COPC have been embraced to varying degrees by medical schools. The family medicine residency review requirements include formal instruction in community medicine, which involves a structured curriculum with didactic and experimental components and participation in clinical experiences such as community resources, public health departments, occupational medicine, community health assessment, community health priorities, and health education programs. Guidelines for excellence developed by the Residency Program Solutions for Family Medicine include a more specific curriculum geared toward population-based solutions to health problems. Additionally, national family medicine leadership groups have recommended that COPC training be a formal part of the curriculum for all residency programs.[27, 28] The Residency Review Committee for Pediatrics also requires instruction and training in community-oriented care, with particular attention to underserved communities and training in the role of health advocate.[29]

Likewise, the Liaison Committee on Medical Education has accreditation requirements for medical schools in the United States and Canada that cover the teaching of prevention, health promotion, cultural competency, and social determinants of disease. These requirements, though not specified as community medicine or COPC, are encompassed by the COPC concept.[30] A number of family medicine programs have included components of the COPC experience as part of their required curricula, such as Mercer University's use of the COPC model to teach students to use community resources for chronic disease management.[31]

In summary, two of the major disciplines in primary care graduate education, as well as allopathic medicine's accrediting body, specifically require the teaching of community medicine or components of COPC.

Challenges of Community-Oriented Primary Care

The challenges imposed by the COPC model have been addressed, in terms of both perceived effectiveness and outcomes for improving the health of a given community.

Cost

One of the most significant issues raised in the United States since the introduction of the COPC concept has been the sustainability of a system with little financial support. In reality, some of COPC's greatest successes have been in the public sector or in partially public-financed health care systems with relatively stable patient populations and external funding sources that are not dependent on the fee-for-service reimbursement system. Some of the more sustainable systems in other countries have occurred where there are alternative funding programs to help cover the extra expenditures in time, resources, and effort.

Phenomenon of inclusion

Mullan and Epstein discuss the "phenomenon of inclusion," which refers to the process of illuminating problems that require special attention.[22] In this sense, COPC can be perceived as placing an extra burden on a medical practice, requiring it to perform more work and do more activities than it had in the past, exhausting the individuals providing the care in the process.

Clarity of terms and methodology

Debates have ensued over the years concerning the COPC methodology. Some advocate strict adherence to the process to ensure a common approach and more predictable results. Others take the more casual view that clinicians should merely have some process that ensures community participation in decision making at some level. This lack of clarity in the definition of COPC is demonstrated by surveys of family medicine residents and faculty, who indicate uncertainty about the core elements of COPC.[32]

The effectiveness of COPC programs has also been debated. Outstanding success stories have been recorded in municipal health systems, such as at Parkland Hospital in Dallas.[26] Evaluations of these COPC programs have revealed shorter hospital stays, improvement in infant mortality rates, and lower costs for patients in the COPC service area compared with other areas, even when accounting for other variables.[27]

Community health interventions in general have had varied degrees of success, partly because of how they are evaluated; for the most part, assessments focus on the individual and not the community. A recent systematic review found no evidence that the COPC model is any more effective than other community health approaches. There appears to be little evidence that strict adherence to the COPC model is necessary to ensure a positive outcome. However, the wrong questions may have been asked when determining what constitutes a positive outcome. A visitor returning to the Karks' Pholela Health Centre years after the disintegration of the original program noted a strong sense of community pride and responsibility that was lacking in similar communities that were not part of the original COPC project. These more subtle measures of success have been difficult to document and quantify. As Gavagan states, the standard methods of conducting research may not have recognized substantial changes in customer satisfaction, community development analysis, health center and community communication, or other long-term health outcomes. Different evaluation methods, such as those introduced by qualitative research, may be necessary to demonstrate these values.[14]

The Future

What is the future of the COPC model? Is it relevant to the practice of medicine in the twenty-first century, and will it have a role in developing a closer working relationship between primary care and public health? It has been widely accepted that health care in the United States is in great need of change. There are serious concerns about the cost of care, the large percentage of uninsured, and the resultant inequities in care. As a whole, the United States experiences less favorable health outcomes than countries that spend considerably less on health care but have other reimbursement and access systems. Beginning in the latter part of the twentieth century, attempts were made to address these concerns. Health maintenance organizations (HMOs) were developed in part to control costs in both the public and private sectors. In general, interest in managed care organizations has waned since the initial flurry of activity, although such organizations are still important in certain sections of the country. In theory, the contractual arrangements of capitated payments should provide some incentive to maintain and improve the health status of a given population; in practice, however, this has been an infrequent occurrence. Community-based programs of disease prevention and health improvement may not show obvious benefits within the time frame of HMO patients' routine enrollment period. Also, it has been difficult to define the target population of an HMO beyond the actual patients in a given practice—the issue of Deuschle's definition of "constituency" as opposed to "community." Funding is also a barrier, since community-based programs have not traditionally been funded by HMOs. Last, the lack of proven efficacy has limited the enthusiasm for the financial investment required, even though many public programs have incorporated the basic components of COPC in their care models.[33]

By 2004, the major family medicine organizations initiated the Future of Family Medicine Project, and one of its key concepts was a "strategy to transform and renew the discipline of family medicine to meet the needs of patients in a changing health care environment." The core values of primary care were reaffirmed to include continuing, compassionate, comprehensive, and personal care *provided within the context of family and community*. This "new" model of care, later known as the patient-centered medical home (PCMH), had first been promulgated by the American Academy of Pediatrics in 1967, and its principles for rejuvenating primary care were affirmed by all the major organizations representing primary care in 2007. As Stange and colleagues define PCMH, it has four components: (1) the four fundamental values of primary care (continuing, compassionate, comprehensive, and personal care), (2) new ways of organizing a practice, (3) development of a practice's internal capabilities, and (4) health care system and reimbursement changes. In elucidating the issues surrounding the last component, they note that a change in primary care providers' reimbursement is essential to the recruitment of an adequate number of health care professionals to provide the needed services; the method of reimbursement will need to change to adequately reward efforts other than "face time" with the provider; and patient participation in decision making is necessary and expected by both patients and providers.[34]

The first PCMH demonstration projects began in 2006, and the evaluators concluded that the institutional changes were much more difficult to implement than previously considered and that a two-year evaluation period was too short to accurately assess the outcomes. Moreover, the evaluators noted that "to meet diverse and comprehensive patient needs, medical homes need to have robust and collaborative relationships with hospitals, nursing homes, specialists, other health care professionals, and community agencies. This integrated neighborhood must appear seamless to the patient."[35] The recent development of accountable care organizations may help address this need.

The PCMH concept is central to the Affordable Care Act of 2010. The availability of health insurance for millions of additional people will bring new challenges to the primary care system. One major change that should help is the improvement in information systems over the past decade. By 2016, $29 billion will be spent on health information technology, with a portion going to aid primary care practices in developing electronic health records. Additionally, advances in geographic information systems are being used in primary care settings and in COPC activities, and these could be more readily available and affordable in the near future.[36] A new appreciation for the value of qualitative information in COPC decision making, such as that obtained from focus groups and key informant studies, could lead to the development of better community opinion information. These advances should help standardize the COPC process and make the activity more approachable and affordable.

In the last several decades, strong evidence has emerged that primary care is crucial to an equitable, affordable, and accountable health care system that controls costs and improves health outcomes. A vibrant primary care system improves the utilization of preventive health services, decreases unnecessary hospitalizations, and improves outcomes through decreased overall mortality and morbidity and increased patient satisfaction. As Phillips and Bazemore note, primary care "is not the solution to every health care problem, but few, if any, health-related problems can be addressed without it."[37]

COPC was first implemented more than seventy years ago, and it has been enthusiastically embraced by many provider groups over the years, despite its lack of adoption throughout the U.S. health care system. It has arguably made a major difference in the health care programs where it has been embraced, particularly for vulnerable populations. It has also been an important concept in educating students about communities, social and cultural aspects of health, and the importance of health care teams. Most important, it has involved community decision making and, in its best renditions, has been bottom-up by design. The newest model of care, the PCMH, has elements of the COPC process embedded in it, even if they are not called by that name, and it provides hope that the renewed focus on the patient, family, and community will transform health care in the United States.

Notes

1. Willard W, chairman. *Meeting the Challenge of Family Practice.* Ad Hoc Committee on Education for Family Practice of the Council on Medical Education, American Medical Association. Chicago: American Medical Association; 1966.

2. Millis JS, chairman. *The Graduate Education of Physicians.* Citizens Commission on Graduate Medical Education. Chicago: American Medical Association; 1966.

3. Donaldson M, Yordy K, Vanselow N. *Primary Care: America's Health in a New Era.* Institute of Medicine. Washington, DC: National Academy Press; 1996:2.

4. Vanselow NA, Donaldson MS. From the Institute of Medicine: A new definition of primary care. *JAMA.* 1995;273(3):192.

5. Friedberg MW, Schneider EC. Primary care: A critical review of the evidence on quality and costs of health care. *Health Aff.* 2010;29(5):766–772.

6. Shi L, Starfield B. Primary care, income inequality, and self-rated health in the United States: A mixed-level analysis. *Int J Health Sci.* 2000;30:541–555.

7. Franks P, Fiscella K. Primary care physicians and specialists as personal physicians: Health care expenditures and mortality experience. *J Fam Pract.* 1998;327:424–429.

8. Regan J, Schempf AH, Yoon J, Politzer RM. The role of federally funded health centers in serving the rural population. *J Rural Health.* 2003;19:117–124.

9. Ryan S, Riley A, Kang M, Starfield B. The effects of regular source of care and health need on medical care use among rural adolescents. *Arch Pediatr Adolesc Med.* 2001;155:184–190.

10. Shi L. Primary care, specialty care, and life chances. *Int J Health Serv.* 1994;24:431–458.

11. Starfield B, Shi L, Macinko J. Contribution of primary care to health systems and health. *Milbank Q.* 2005;83(3):457–502.

12. Deuschle K. Interview by Richard Smoot. University of Kentucky Medical Center Oral History Project. August 20, 1987.

13. Tapp JW, Deuschle KW. The community medicine clerkship: A guide for teachers and students of community medicine. *Milbank Q.* 1969;48(4):411–447.

14. Gavagan T. A systematic review of COPC: Evidence for effectiveness. *J Health Care Poor Underserved.* 2008;19(3):963–980.

15. Tollman SM. The Pholela Health Centre—the origins of community-oriented primary care (COPC). *South African Med J.* 1994;10:653–658.

16. King's Fund. *Community-Oriented Primary Care: A Resource for Developers.* London: King Edward's Hospital Fund for London; 1994.

17. Epstein L, Gofin J, Gofin R, Neumark Y. The Jerusalem experience: Three decades of service, research, and training in community-oriented primary care. *Am J Public Health.* 2002;11:1717–1721.

18. Madison DL, Shenkin BN. *Leadership for Community-Responsive Practice: Report to the Bureau of Health Manpower by the Rural Practice Project Team.* Chapel Hill, NC: Bureau of Health Manpower; 1978.

19. Deuschle K. Community-oriented primary care: Lessons learned in three decades. *J Community Health.* 1982;8(1):13–22.

20. Abramson JH. Community-oriented primary care—strategy, approaches, and practice: A review. *Public Health Rev.* 1988;16:35–98.

21. Nutting PA, Connor EM. *Community Oriented Primary Care: A Practical Assessment.* Vol. 1. Institute of Medicine. Washington, DC: National Academy Press; 1984.

22. Mullan F, Epstein L. Community-oriented primary care: New relevance in a changing world. *Am J Public Health.* 2002;92(11):1748–1755.

23. Dresang LT, Brebrick L, Murray D, Shallue A, Sullivan-Vedder L. Family medicine in Cuba: Community-oriented primary care and complementary and alternative medicine. *J Am Board Fam Pract.* 2005;18:297–303.

24. Gofin J, Foz G. Training and application of community-oriented primary care (COPC) through family medicine in Catalonia, Spain. *Fam Med.* 2008;40(3):196–202.

25. Geiger H. The meaning of community oriented primary care in the American context. In: *Community Oriented Primary Care: New Directions for Health Service Delivery.* Division of Health Care Services, Institute of Medicine. Washington, DC: National Academy Press; 1983:60–90.

26. Pickens S, Boumbulian P, Anderson R, Ross S, Phillips S. Community-oriented primary care in action: A Dallas story. *Am J Public Health.* 2002;92(11):1728–1732.

27. Plescia M, Konen JC, Lincourt A. The state of community medicine training in family practice residency programs. *Fam Med.* 2002;34(3):177–182.

28. Accreditation Council for Graduate Medical Education. Family Medicine Program Requirements. July 2007. http://www.acgme.org/acWebsite/RRC_120/120_prIndex.asp. Accessed August 9, 2011.

29. Pediatrics Program Requirements. July 2007. http://www.acgme.org/acWebsite/RRC_320/320_prIndex.asp. Accessed August 9, 2011.

30. Liaison Committee on Medical Education. Functions and Structure of a Medical School: Standards for Accreditation of Medical Education Programs Leading to the M.D. Degree. 2011. http://www.lcme.org/functions2011may.pdf. Accessed August 9, 2011.

31. Dent MM, Mathis MW, Outland M, McKinley T, Industrious D. Chronic

disease management: Teaching medical students to incorporate community. *Fam Med.* 2010;42(10):736–740.

32. Williams R, Foldy S. The state of community-oriented primary care: Physician and residency program surveys. *Fam Med.* 1994;26(4):232–237.

33. Lairson DR, Schulmeier G, Begley CE, Aday LA, Slater CH. Managed care and community-oriented care: Conflict or complement? *J Health Care Poor Underserved.* 1997;8(1):36–55.

34. Stange K, et al. Defining and measuring the patient-centered medical home. *J Gen Intern Med.* 2010;25(6):601–612.

35. Nutting P, Crabtree B, Miller W, Stange K, Stewart E, Jaén C. Transforming physician practices to patient-centered medical homes: Lessons from the National Demonstration Project. *Health.* 2011;30(3):439–445.

36. Bazemore A, Phillips R, Miyoshi T. Harnessing geographic information systems (GIS) to enable community-oriented primary care. *J Am Board Fam Med.* 2010;23(1):22–31.

37. Phillips R, Bazemore A. Primary care and why it matters for U.S. health system reform. *Health Aff.* 2010;29(5):806–810.

5

Who Is the Public in Public Health?

David Mathews

Public health is a common term, but few individuals think about its meaning. People understand that the *health* portion of the term includes immunizations, restaurant inspections, and water quality reports. The *public* portion of the term encompasses everyone—all Americans—and anything that is for the good of all. Is the *public* in *public health* like the *public* in *public restrooms* or *public transportation*—something open and accessible to anyone? Public health practitioners may disagree. A better analogy may be the *public* in *public education*. But the more a definition is sought, the less obvious the meaning becomes.

This chapter is based on Kettering Foundation research, which focuses on democracy, not public health. As such, it is worthwhile to raise the question of whether the *public* in *public health* has any relation to the *public* in a democratic, not just a demographic, sense. The pursuit of this question could add a new dimension to the field of public health and might lead to practical insights that practitioners could use in their efforts to engage citizens and their communities.

A democratic understanding of the public puts a spotlight on the relationship between communities and the health of the people who live in them. This is an important relationship; the norms in a community affect the behavior of residents and have a bearing on the illnesses tied to behavior. Success in changing behavior is determined by the way a community goes about it. The means of changing behavior include the practices citizens use to solve problems, including problems that lead to illness.

Citizens in communities that are adept at solving their problems use distinctive practices that allow them to act together and wisely, which is to say, democratically. However, the routines that public health practitioners follow in doing their work may not align productively with the practices citizens use in doing theirs. When public health practitioners go about their work as they should, sometimes this unintentionally interferes with the work citizens perform—work that can help solve the problems that undermine the public's health. This chapter focuses on how to better align professional routines with the various practices citizens use in democratic problem solving, with the hope of sparking new insights that public health practitioners can turn into useful innovations.

To think of the public in a democratic context immediately raises a question: what is a democracy? *Democracy* has a number of valid definitions. For some, it is a form of government based on majority rule. It can also be a political system that promotes justice and equity or a way of life that encourages respect and freedom of association.[1] In its research, Kettering uses something close to the ancient Greek concept of democracy, which locates sovereignty and legitimate power, or control, in the people—or what the Pilgrims called a "civic body politic." Citizens use this power to rule themselves and shape their future.

A certain logic follows from this premise. Sovereign monarchs exercise power by utilizing the power to act. So it follows that the sovereign citizenry is a collective political actor, a producer rather than a beneficiary or a constituency; it is not a dependent body to be acted for or upon. A sovereign citizenry acts together to produce things that serve the good of all. And the things people produce by working with others—public goods—bring about change, which is what having power or control means. Public goods are made through public or civic work—that is, work done by citizens joining forces.[2] Historically, the things citizens make have included schools, hospitals, and even the country itself. Today, the products of citizens' collective efforts—their civic work—range from campaigns that get drunk drivers off the road to neighborhood watches that make communities safer.

The importance of what citizens can do with other citizens is particularly evident following natural disasters, according to scholars such as Monica Schoch-Spana. Research shows that in the first days after a disaster, survival depends largely on the resilience of communities. As Schoch-Spana and her colleagues explain: "Successful remedies and recovery for communitywide disasters are neither conceived nor implemented solely by trained emergency personnel, nor are they confined to preauthorized procedures. Family members, friends, coworkers, neighbors, and strangers who happen to be in the vicinity often carry out search and rescue activities and provide medical aid before police, fire, and other officials even arrive on the scene. In epidemics, volunteers have helped conduct mass vaccination campaigns, nurse homebound patients, and meet the broad social needs of sick people and their families." Unfortunately, these scholars found that practitioners were not always receptive to citizens' contributions: "Some emergency authorities also have mistakenly interpreted citizen-led interventions in past and present disasters as evidence of failure on the part of responders. In reality, government leaders, public health and safety professionals, and communities at-large have complementary and mutually supportive roles to play in mass emergencies."[3]

Nobel Prize winner Elinor Ostrom has demonstrated that the things citizens make can reinforce what institutions and their professionals produce. Her research on *coproduction* implies that unless the institutions that provide health care have the benefit of public goods, they cannot possibly provide all that a healthy nation requires.[4] For instance, the work of citizens has been critical in combating the social forces that contribute to illnesses. Using evidence from a health project in Finland, Milstein at the Centers for Disease Control and Prevention (CDC) has shown that citizen initiatives can reduce the incidence of illnesses, such as heart disease, stroke, and lung cancer, which result in hospitalization.[5]

Examples of Citizens Deliberating and Acting

Before explaining democratic practices, a review of a case involving a community with an air pollution problem—a problem that can polarize and immobilize a political system—will be helpful. The community was located in a hub of the automotive industry, and people there depended on the manufacture of cars, which produced much of the pollution. Efforts to control air pollution easily could have pitted car manufacturers against environmentalists. Such disputes usually result in lengthy litigation, while air quality continues to deteriorate.

In this case, however, a public health official encouraged a democratic practice, deliberative decision making, which helped depolarize the issue. Rather than holding the usual public meetings, a member of the local health department attended numerous small meetings. Instead of attempting to educate citizens or help them reach an agreed-on solution, the official assisted them in talking to one another by creating a framework for their meetings. To prompt public deliberation on the pros and cons of the issue, rather than a debate, major options for dealing with air quality were considered, and forum participants weighed the advantages and disadvantages of each one. For instance, stricter emission standards would reduce pollutants but also make cars costlier and thus less competitive in the marketplace. As they struggled with what was obviously a difficult decision, citizens came to see the issue in several dimensions. Although they did not agree on one particular solution, they were less susceptible to being polarized. When citizens come to appreciate the complexity of an issue, officials have greater latitude to move ahead in addressing it, even though the issue may be a political third rail (too hot to touch).[6]

The CDC has also used public deliberation when developing policies for pandemic flu outbreaks. For instance, difficult decisions have to be made concerning how to allocate the initial supply of vaccines. Rather than relying on polls and interviews, CDC officials joined with civic organizations to determine what people think when confronted with difficult choices: would they try to protect society as a whole, or only the most vulnerable? (The research found that citizens consistently cited protecting society as the top priority.)[7]

In both cases, health officials selected issues in which a sovereign public should have a voice. Public health officials did not expect citizens to make the same decisions that practitioners would make, such as how best to implement policies; nor did they expect the public's decisions to be based on technical and scientific expertise.

In other situations, citizens must do more than respond to policy options. They must act themselves, and their actions have to produce the things needed to solve the problem. This civic work might result in a community program that encourages people to lose weight or in a volunteer corps to check on the elderly during a summer heat wave. The projects may vary, but they create public goods that benefit the community as a whole. The real challenge is not polarization but disagreements over the right thing to do. People may agree that there is a problem in the community, but they may disagree on what it is or what should be done about it. These disagreements stand in the way of people joining forces and working together.

Democratic self-organizing, despite its long history, does not always occur, and when it does not, public health practitioners may be tempted to rush in. However, what they do should not preclude self-organizing. Perhaps their assistance should be more diagnostic than didactic, more coaching than directing, more building on what grows than mobilizing for new projects. Such actions would be consistent with self-organizing and self-rule.

Democratic Practices

The way citizens conduct civic work might be called *democratic practices. Practices* are different from purely instrumental *techniques*, a distinction made by the ancient Greeks. This difference is subtle yet crucial, particularly given today's multitude of techniques for facilitating meetings and planning. There is nothing wrong with techniques, but unlike practices, they do not possess moral value. For example, hammering is a carpenter's technique; its only benefit is driving a nail, although a degree of skill is involved. Practices are different; they are not a set of skills to be taught. Democratic practices express the virtues associated with democracy—good judgment, cooperation, social responsibility. They can be cultivated, and they are sources of moral energy that generate political will and the commitments needed to drive civic work.

To date, Kettering's research has identified six practices used in the work citizens do with citizens: naming, framing, deliberative decision making, identifying and committing resources, organizing complementary acting, and public learning. These practices are elements in a theory of democracy that have everyday applications in the life of a community. They are democratic, in that they increase the control people have over their future. For each practice, there are differences between what occurs in civic work and the routines usually followed by public health practitioners. Neither is better than the other, and their differences are appropriate. The confusion between professional routines and democratic practices occurs because both accomplish similar work, and the tasks are usually identical. Politics, democratic or not, involves identifying and solving problems. Decisions have to be made along the way, and after a course of action is determined, resources must be located and deployed. The results should always be assessed. *How* such things are accomplished determines whether they are democratic. The greatest misalignment of professional routines and democratic practices occurs when both public health practitioners and citizens are trying to accomplish the same tasks, but there is a failure to recognize the differences in *how* they go about it.

Naming

The first practice involves identifying or describing a problem and selecting the terms to be used. It begins when something has happened—for instance, the local economy has collapsed—and people talk about how they and their families are affected. Citizens see problems in terms of what is most valuable to them, and when they name problems to capture what they hold dear, the naming takes on a democratic coloration. Professional names, in contrast, tend to reflect professional expertise.

Framing

The second practice has to do with what citizens think should be done about a problem, which follows from their conception of it. People propose various options for dealing with a problem, depending on what is most valuable to them, and each option has advantages and disadvantages. When all the major

options have been identified, and their pros and cons have been fairly presented, a democratic framework for decision making is created. Recognizing that
every option has advantages as well as disadvantages also exposes the tensions
that have to be worked through. Public health practitioners create frameworks
for decision making as well, but their options are typically based on technical
feasibility and the weight of scientific evidence.

Deliberative decision making

The third practice is determining which option is best. When people make
decisions by weighing the options against all that they value, they deliberate.
Public health practitioners also make decisions, and they are not indifferent to
the things citizens value, but they are more likely to weigh hard evidence rather than deal with intangibles.

Identifying and committing resources

The fourth practice involves identifying the resources needed to solve a problem and obtaining commitments to use them. Civic resources are assets found
in the experiences and talents of people.[8] Typically, they are less tangible than
professional resources and cannot be commandeered. They have to be committed through the mutual promises people make to one another.

Organizing complementary acting

Ideally, the actions decided on during public deliberations complement one
another. If so, the power of what citizens do increases due to mutual reinforcement; the whole of their effort becomes greater than the sum of the parts. Professional action tends to be uniform and based on a single plan, whereas civic
action varies by the number of civic actors and is more orchestrated than organized, more strategically opportunistic than directed by a plan.

Public learning

Public learning is not a separate practice but rather something that occurs
throughout the work of citizens. It is the most important practice of all because it provides the momentum to keep the work moving ahead on the
most difficult problems, those that defy professional expertise and persist
despite institutional efforts to eradicate them. Public health practitioners
learn by comparing results to fixed goals; citizens are more likely to learn

by reassessing what is most valuable, as well as through the results of collective efforts.

The practices that result in citizens doing things that contribute to public health may seem somewhat removed from the problems public health practitioners face every day, particularly if they are frustrated in their efforts to involve people in their communities. Complaints from professionals in various fields include the following:

1. People are apathetic; they do not respond when asked to become involved. Corporate interests tend to dominate the community.
2. Citizens do not trust one another and are more likely to disagree than to work together. They may even be afraid of one another, and they do not trust the systems practitioners work in.
3. If citizens do become interested in an issue, they are usually just emotionally involved and make ill-advised decisions.
4. There is really not much people can do, as they do not have the resources.
5. Even if people promise to do something together, many will not show up, and there is no way to enforce what they promised.
6. People are too disorganized to be effective; everyone wants to go his or her own way.
7. Even when a civic project gets started, it often stops because the momentum is easily lost.
8. There is no way to tell whether a civic project has been effective; citizens seldom evaluate objectively.

Professionals are not imagining these problems; they are real and, to some degree, unavoidable. Democratic practices can serve as a counterforce: Naming problems in terms of the things citizens care deeply about engages them. Framing problems to bring out tensions and disagreements assists citizens in working through them. Deliberative decision making increases the possibility that the public's judgment will be sound, countering polarization. Such decision making enriches people's understanding of a problem, helping them to recognize untapped resources. Commitments to use these resources can be enforced by the covenants people make with one another when legal contracts are inappropriate. Although deliberative decision making may not end in total agreement, it can result in a common sense of purpose and direction that allows civic initiatives to complement one another with a minimum of coordination. Learning throughout civic work not only maintains the momentum but also fosters evaluations that go deeper than conventional assessments of results.

Suggsville: Democratic Practices in Everyday Life

Opportunities to encourage democratic practices and to better align professional work with civic work occur every day; the key is to recognize them. Seizing these opportunities may not require public health practitioners to do more or different work but rather to work in a different way. For instance, although public health practitioners may be required to hold public meetings (as in the air pollution case), they can encourage public deliberation rather than discussion and debate.

To show where opportunities to develop democratic practices occur every day, the Kettering Foundation has created a composite town called Suggsville, based on observations in scores of real communities.[9] The Suggsville composite is based on places with less-than-ideal conditions, to emphasize the difficulties citizens encounter in doing their work. The Suggsville story is not exclusively about health, but health problems are closely connected with an array of other problems. In democratic problem solving, the practices used are the same, whatever the issues. Professionals in one field would be well served if their efforts to foster civic work were matched by efforts in other fields.

Naming problems to capture what is most valuable to citizens

Suggsville was rural and poor. Once a prosperous farming community, the town began to decline during the 1970s as the agricultural economy floundered. By the 1990s, the unemployment rate soared above 40 percent. Property values plummeted. With little else to replace the income from idle farms, a drug trade flourished. A majority of Suggsville's children were born to single teenagers. The schools were plagued with low test scores and high dropout rates. Not surprisingly, disease rates were higher than in most communities. The most common illnesses were diabetes, heart disease, and cancer. But obesity was becoming epidemic, and alcoholism was pervasive. Everyone who could leave the town had done so, especially college-educated young adults. Making matters worse, the community was sharply divided: rich and poor, black and white.

During informal encounters after church services, Suggsvillians patronizing the one grocery store that survived discussed what was happening with friends and neighbors. Different groups made small talk and mulled over the town's difficulties. No decisions were made, and no actions were taken. Then a group of professionals from a nearby university, which had been consulting on the town's problems, suggested that Suggsvillians meet, assess their situation, and decide what they might do. Initially, the university's proposal for a town meeting drew the predictable handful. People sat in racially homogeneous clusters—until someone rearranged the chairs in a circle and citizens began to mingle. After participants got off their favorite soapboxes, told their own stories, and looked for others to blame, they settled down to identifying the problems that concerned everyone. Economic security was at the top of the list, but it wasn't the only concern. Crime was another.

The Suggsville conversation was an opportunity to develop a democratic practice. People could name their problems in terms that resonated with the things they valued.[10] Determining what people consider valuable is not difficult. However, naming a problem in terms of what people hold dear requires more than simply describing it in everyday language. When people talk about what is at stake, they bring up concerns that are deeply important to almost everyone—to be safe from danger, to be secure from economic privation, to be free to pursue their own interests, and to be treated fairly by others. These collective motives are counterparts to the individual needs that Abraham Maslow found to be common among all human beings. They are more fundamental than the interests that grow out of our particular circumstances (which may change). They are different from values, which vary in importance, depending on our circumstances.

Some individual needs are quite tangible, such as food; others are intangible, such as being loved. The same is true of collective needs. One community that Kettering observed was facing corruption in high places and egregious crimes on the streets. Citizens asked themselves what they valued most, and virtually everyone said that, more than anything else, they wanted to live in a place that made them proud. Pride is an intangible aspiration rarely mentioned in planning documents or lists of goals. Still, the need to be proud of a city is a powerful political imperative.

This distinction and its implications for public health practitioners are illustrated in Wendell Berry's story of an economist who told farmers that it was cheaper to rent land than to buy it, which was factually correct at the time. One farmer responded, however, by telling the economist that his forebears did not come to America to be renters.[11] Something else of value to the farmers, other than profits, was at stake.

As noted earlier, the terms people use to describe problems are different from those practitioners use. The names that practitioners give issues, though technically accurate, often exclude the more subjective values people associate with issues. The unfortunate result is that people do not necessarily feel any connection to issues that practitioners see as important, and this lack of connection may be interpreted as indifference on the part of the public.

Professional names can also suggest that there is little citizens can do about a problem except to support practitioners and the institutions where they work. Consequently, people are disinclined to become involved because they do not see how they can make a difference. For instance, when public health departments invite citizens to participate in solving a problem, the invitation may sound hollow because of the way the problem has been framed. Professionals in all fields worry about apathetic citizens, but naming problems in public terms facilitates the work of citizens, since the names people use encourage them to own their problems, and owning problems is a potent source of energy for civic work.

Framing issues to identify all the options

As the town meetings continued, Suggsvillians laid out a number of concerns reflecting the things they valued. People didn't choose just one name and discard all the others. The economy was just the first name for the town's problem, and it resonated with concerns about security. Then people identified other problems, such as family instability and an increase in drug abuse. These, too, touched different notions of security that citizens held dear.

Not coincidentally, as people in Suggsville added names to their problems, they tended to implicate themselves in solving them. They could do something about the alcoholism that was threatening both families and the social order, and they could do something about the children who suffered when adults took little responsibility for their well-being.

Given concerns about the economy, one of the first proposals was to recruit a manufacturing company to build a plant in the town. No one rejected the suggestion; it stayed on the table. However, some participants in the conversations had a practical objection—every other town was competing for new industries, and some development authorities recommended a grow-your-own business strategy. Not convinced that this was a good recommendation, the few who still felt strongly about recruiting a new industry left the group and went to the state office of economic development for assistance. Nonetheless, the majority of the participants continued to discuss what might be done to support local businesses. Several mentioned a restaurant that had opened recently; it seemed to have the potential to stimulate a modest revival of the downtown area. Unfortunately, that potential wasn't being realized because unemployed men (and youngsters who liked to hang out with them) were congregating on the street in front of the restaurant and drinking. Customers shied away.

Notice what was happening in the Suggsville meetings. At this point, the group was proposing possible courses of action to revive the economy. Indeed, almost everyone assumed that the problem was the economy, but that was beginning to change as other concerns suggested additional courses of action. No one was ready to delve into the pros and cons of the various proposals, beyond noting that they all had advantages and disadvantages. Hearing everyone's vision of Suggsville's future was an opportunity to create a comprehensive and democratic framework for the decisions that needed to be made about how to make those visions a reality.

Issues are constantly being framed in communities by the media and by officeholders. Sometimes an issue is framed around a single plan of action; this framework tells citizens to take it or leave it. Another common framework pits two possible solutions against each other and encourages a debate between advocates. Neither of these frameworks promotes the kind of deliberation that leads to civic work. Public decision making is better served by a framework that includes all the major options (usually three or four) and also identifies the tensions among the things people consider valuable, which are embedded in the options. As already noted, recognizing these tensions is key to dealing with disagreements.

As people wrestle with the task of figuring out what their community should do, they find themselves pulled in different directions. They want to do something that reinforces what they value without losing or compromising something equally important. People often face tensions like these in their personal and public lives. Even things that are universally valued, such as freedom and security, can be in conflict. Under certain circumstances, providing more security can impinge on personal freedom, and people differ on how much freedom they are willing to sacrifice in order to increase their security. These differences are evident when it comes to addressing the threat from terrorism.

Why emphasize tensions and run the risk of provoking disputes when the political environment already suffers from partisan rancor and incivility? Tensions invariably arouse strong feelings, and nothing can make those emotions disappear. However, if the framing begins by recognizing what citizens value, people may realize that they differ over the means to achieve the same ends. For instance, security and freedom are valued by everyone, but individuals may differ on how to balance the two.

Recognizing tensions among citizens also makes people more aware of the tensions within themselves. When individuals realize that they are pulled in different directions personally, they tend to be less absolute in their opinions and more open to the views of others, even those with whom they disagree. This openness allows individuals to see problems from different perspectives. The result is that there is a more complete view of the problem, and this enlarged sense is crucial to effective problem solving. As people work through tensions by accepting trade-offs, they often reach a point where the whole community can move ahead and deal with a problem.[12] A sense of which actions are or are not likely to be supported is enough, since complete agreement is rare.

If framing is key to dealing with disagreements, how does it occur in real time? One simple question can start the process: if you are *that* concerned, what do you think should be done? As happened in Suggsville, people usually respond by talking about both their concerns and the actions they favor. Typically, the concerns are implicit in the suggestions for action.

People's concerns (and there are usually many) generate a variety of specific proposals for action. For instance, if Suggsville were hit by a rash of burglaries, most people would be concerned about their physical safety, which is surely a basic political motive. Some would want more police visible on the streets. Others might favor a neighborhood watch. Even though these actions are different, they both center around one basic concern—safety. In that sense, they are two parts of one option, which might be characterized as protection through surveillance. An option is made up of actions that have the same purpose or move in the same direction.

A framework that recognizes all the relevant concerns and lays out all the main options for addressing them, along with the various actions and actors that must be involved, sets the stage for a fair trial. For a trial to be truly fair, each option has to be presented with its best foot forward, and all its drawbacks have to be considered as well. Fairness is particularly important when public health practitioners encounter polarizing issues such as disposing of hazardous materials or distributing vaccines.

Deliberating publicly to make sound decisions

At the next Suggsville town meeting, attendance was higher, and people started talking about what could be done to save the restaurant.

The police chief argued that the problem was loitering and recommended stricter enforcement of ordinances. In the chief's opinion, the downsides to strict law enforcement were less serious than the loitering itself. Others were not so sure. Strict enforcement, even if it worked to clear the streets, might give the community the feel of a police state. This was a tension to be worked through. Still others worried about the problems that contributed to loitering. One woman suggested that loitering was symptomatic of widespread alcoholism.

As citizens put their concerns on the table, they struggled with what was most important to the welfare of the community. People valued a great many things. The Suggsville they hoped to create would be family friendly and safe for kids. It would have good schools as well as a good economy. Yet everything that had to be done to reach these objectives had potential downsides. Tensions were unavoidable. People were ready to weigh the potential consequences of different options because they had to decide what was most valuable to the community.

Step outside Suggsville again and consider the opportunity to turn a discussion into a democratic practice, a public deliberation. The door is open to raise questions: if citizens do what an individual suggests—and it works, but it also has negative consequences—will that person still stand by his proposal? Deliberating helps the citizenry move from initial reactions and hastily formed opinions to a more shared and reflective judgment. Whether the decisions made are wise cannot be known until results are observed. Nonetheless, decisions are more likely to be sound if the course of action chosen is consistent with what is believed to be most important for the well-being of all. Perhaps this is why the ancient Greeks defined deliberation as the talk used to teach before any action occurs.[13] Of course, public judgments may eventually prove faulty, since the voice of the people is not infallible.

Public health practitioners can benefit from examining how deliberation functions. First of all, a deliberative framework brings people face-to-face with the tensions involved in choosing among options that have both positive and negative consequences. Citizens deliberate to work through the tensions that exist both within and among options. This work—choice work—does not occur all at once; it occurs in stages, and these stages have important implications for practitioners.[14] Knowing where citizens are—and are not—in their thinking is crucial in engaging them.

Initially, citizens may not even be sure there is an issue they should be concerned about. Perhaps it seems that nothing dear to them is at stake. Later, they may become aware of a problem that touches on something they value, but they simply complain about it. The "issue" is one of who to blame. At this stage, people may not see the tensions or the necessity to act. If the tensions do become apparent, people usually struggle as they weigh the advantages and disadvantages of various options. Eventually, citizens may work through an issue and settle on a range of actions that move in a common direction.

Consider what these stages suggest for civic engagement strategies. When citizens are not yet sure a problem exists, professionals may be well advised to start where people start, even though the professionals may have moved on in their thinking. Citizens are not ready to consider solutions at this point. The question that has to be addressed is, what is the issue? When people recognize that there is a serious issue yet look for a scapegoat, again, revisiting the nature of the problem seems more likely to be successful than promoting a solution. Even when citizens move past blaming, they may still be unsure what their options are and what trade-offs they will have to make. If so, they are very susceptible to being polarized, particularly if professionals or politicians engage in a hard-sell strategy. However, once people reach the point of struggling with trade-offs, they are more likely to be open to information that is relevant to their concerns.

For public health practitioners, the implications of these stages are rather clear. For instance, providing factual information from experts is important, but it cannot substitute for the deliberating people must do to make decisions. The reason is that there are significant differences in the way citizens and professionals go about informing their decisions. In the first place, each group makes different types of decisions. Professionals have to decide what is factual and feasible. Citizens in a democracy have the final say about what *should be.* Professionals decide what to do by consulting evidence produced through rigorous scientific analysis; this evidence distinguishes fact from fiction. When citizens decide what *should be,* they are dealing with moral or normative matters that require sound judgment (there are no experts on moral issues). Citizens inform their judgment by weighing options for solving a problem against all they value or hold dear. The knowledge they use in making a decision comes from comparing their experiences in the cauldron of deliberation. This is socially constructed knowledge that relies on the human faculty for judgment. Facts are essential in making sound decisions, but they are not sufficient.

When citizens finally settle on a general direction, professionals do not have a set of orders they must carry out, but they should have a clear sense of what is and is not supportable. In some cases, professionals believe the best course of action is outside that which is politically permissible. In such cases, public deliberations can tell professionals how the citizenry went about making up its mind, so professionals can engage this thinking when they believe the public has erred.

Although deliberating is difficult and benefits from preparation, it does not require special skills; it is a natural act. Citizens deliberate with family and friends on personal matters all the time. People are attracted to deliberative decision making because their experiences and concerns count as much as professional expertise and data. Public deliberation cannot be for experts only and still be a democratic practice.

Identifying and committing resources

In Suggsville, as people worked through tensions, they turned to implementing their decisions. For instance, some worried that there were too many youngsters with too little adult supervision. In response, several community members proposed things they were willing to do if others would join them: organize baseball and softball leagues, provide after-school classes, expand youth services in the churches, form a band. The observation that alcoholism was contributing to the town's difficulties prompted someone to propose that a chapter of Alcoholics Anonymous be established. Where would it meet? Someone offered a vacant building free of charge. As more projects developed and citizens called on other citizens to join them, new recruits began to attend the meetings. Rather than deciding on a single plan, people mounted an array of initiatives that were loosely coordinated because they were all consistent with the sense of direction emerging from the deliberations.

The naming, framing, and deliberating in Suggsville would be of little consequence unless action followed. Decisions have to be implemented, and that requires identifying and committing resources. Even though citizens have resources that can reinforce institutions and benefit communities, they often go unrecognized and unused. Opportunities to identify these resources occur during deliberations as citizens enlarge their understanding of a problem. When people see a problem more completely, resources that were unrecognized or seemed irrelevant take on new significance. The same is true of the people and organizations that control these resources. Suggsvillians who knew how to coach youngsters in baseball and softball were not an asset until community revitalization was seen as more than a strictly economic problem. Unfortunately, institutional and professional routines can overlook such resources because they do not look like institutional resources. Civic resources are often intangible or are based on personal experiences and skills.

Actually, recognition of these resources can be prompted early on, during framing, by including citizens in the list of potential actors. Institutions—governments, schools, hospitals, and major nongovernmental organizations—are obvious and necessary actors, but they are seldom enough to deal with a community's most persistent problems. These problems have many sources, and the citizenry throughout a community must act.

The difficulty in many cases is that local institutions do not take advantage of the work citizens do with citizens. After citizens have deliberated over an issue and made decisions about what should be done, politics as usual takes over. When it comes to implementation, citizens are pushed to the sidelines. Institutions may acknowledge what people have decided but fall back on familiar routines, such as planning. Some professionals assume that once the people have spoken, it is time for professionals to follow up with institutional resources. Institutional plans do not normally include provisions for civic work.

One reason planning overlooks the work that citizens do with citizens is that institutions are not sure they can count on people to produce. Institutions have money and legal authority; they can rely on enforceable contracts. The democratic public cannot command people or deploy equipment, and it seldom has any legal authority. So why do people do things like organizing patrols on crime-ridden streets when there is no financial inducement or legal obligation? Battling street crime is not just time-consuming; it is dangerous. Most people do what they have pledged to do—in public—because their fellow citizens expect it of them. These commitments are often reciprocal; one group promises, we will do thus and so, if you will do thus and so.

Public covenants may sound idealistic, yet they work. They have their own kind of social or peer group leverage.[15] A community leader explained the generally high attendance at the Suggsville meetings this way: "If you don't show up, somebody will say something to you about it." As in Suggsville, it is not uncommon for deliberations to be followed by mutual promises, either at forums or at subsequent meetings.

Organizing complementary acting

As Suggsville's revival progressed, several people returned to the argument that while encouraging local businesses was fine, this would never provide enough jobs to revive the economy. The town still had to attract outside investment, they insisted. Someone quickly pointed out that the center of town, especially the park, was so unsightly that no one of sound mind would consider Suggsville an attractive site for a new business. Even though some saw little connection between the condition of the park and the ability to recruit industry, no one denied that the town needed a facelift. Suggsville's three-member sanitation crew, however, had all it could do to keep up with garbage collection. Did people feel strongly enough about the cleanup to accept the consequences? Would they show up to clean the park themselves? In the past, the response to similar calls had varied from substantial to minimal. This time, after one of the community forums, a group of people committed to gathering at the park the following Saturday with rakes, mowers, and trash bags.

During most of these meetings, the recently elected mayor sat quietly, keeping an eye on what was happening. The forums had begun during his predecessor's administration, and the town's new leader felt no obligation to the participants. In fact, he was a bit suspicious of what they were doing. Members of the town council believed that the public meetings would result in just another pressure group, or they thought that once the citizens had identified needs, they should step aside and let local agencies take over. No one made any demands on the town government, although some citizens thought it strange that the mayor hadn't offered to help with the cleanup. But before Saturday arrived, people were surprised to find that the mayor had sent the town's garbage crew to the park with trucks and other heavy equipment to do what the tools brought from home could not.

Just as the public has its own distinctive way of moving from decision to action, it has its own distinctive way of acting and organizing action. Government agencies act on behalf of the public, and people act individually by volunteering for all sorts of civic projects. Both are beneficial, but neither constitutes the public acting. Opportunities for the entire citizenry to act occur once people decide on common directions and purposes, as happened in Suggsville.

The public acts in various ways that are organized to reinforce one another when they move in the same direction or serve the same objective. Setting directions and objectives can occur during public deliberation. The result is complementary acting by citizens. Complementary acting is more than cooperation among civic groups; it is not only multifaceted but also mutually reinforcing. Consequently, this way of acting can be coherent without being bureaucratically coordinated. This means that the cost of getting things done is usually lower than if institutional costs were involved. Even though complementary acting requires a degree of coordination (for example, everyone should show up on the same day to clean the park), it is not administratively regulated and does not have administrative expenses.

The payoff from complementary acting goes beyond the concrete products of civic work. Researchers have found that the work people do together, such as cleaning up a park, is valued not just because the park is nicer but also because it demonstrates that people joining forces can make a difference. Working together also builds trust. When people work together, they have a more realistic sense of what they can expect from one another. This is political trust, which is not quite the same as personal trust and should not be confused with it. Political trust can develop among people who are not family or friends. All that is necessary is for citizens to recognize that they need one another to solve their community's problems.

To repeat: complementary public acting supplements institutional action; it is not a substitute for it. This fact has long been recognized in research on urban reform. For instance, Clarence Stone reports that citizens in poorer neighborhoods formed alliances that accomplished far more than any institutions could alone.[16] Professionals have little difficulty in encouraging this type of acting when they value and make a place for it.

Learning as a community

Over the next two years, the ad hoc group that cleaned up the park organized into a more formal civic association. New industry didn't come to Suggsville, although the restaurant held its own. Drugs continued to be a problem, but people's vigilance, together with more surveillance by the police department, reduced the drug trade. The crowds loitering on the streets dwindled away. Alcoholism remained a problem, but more people attended AA meetings. A new summer recreation program became popular with young people, and teenage pregnancies decreased a bit, as did the high school dropout rate.

The community group also took on new issues. For example, local health professionals organized forums on another serious problem: the alarming incidence of breast cancer. Deliberations on how to combat this problem resulted in 20 percent more cancer screenings in one year, which greatly improved the chances for an eventual drop in cancer deaths. Working together on this problem also improved race relations.[17]

As the ad hoc Suggsville improvement group became an official civic association, it experienced the usual internal disputes that detracted from community problem solving. Still, when a controversy was brewing or an emerging issue needed to be addressed, people turned to the association for help. As might be expected, some of the projects didn't work. Fortunately, in most cases, association members adjusted their sights and launched more initiatives. Perhaps this momentum had something to do with the way the association involved the community in the evaluation of projects. The association regularly convened meetings where citizens could reflect on what they had learned, regardless of whether the projects had succeeded. Success wasn't as important as the lessons that could be used in future projects.

Like all six of the democratic practices, community or public learning is a variation on a normal routine (evaluating), yet it is quite distinctive. Unlike traditional evaluations, public learning can supplement the outcome-based assessments that are often used in institutions. In public learning, the citizenry or community itself learns, and the learning is reflected in changed behavior. In other words, the unit of learning is the community, and the measure of learning is community change.

There are obviously many opportunities for a citizenry to learn after a community has acted on a problem. Everyone wants to know whether the effort succeeded. The press declares the results to be beneficial, harmful, or inconsequential. One-on-one conversations bubble up at the supermarket. Outside evaluators make "objective" assessments. The citizenry, however, may not learn a great deal from the media's conclusions, chance conversations, or professional evaluations. One reason is that conventional evaluations unintentionally interfere. For citizens to learn, people have to focus on themselves as a community. The evaluation cannot be limited to what a project has achieved; it has to include how well the citizens worked together. People have to unpack their motives and experiences in order to learn from one another.

Opportunities for public learning are not confined to final evaluations; they can occur during all six practices. To name an issue in public terms is to learn what others value. To frame an issue is to learn about all the options for action—as well as the tensions that need to be worked through. To decide deliberatively is to learn which actions are consistent or inconsistent with what is held most valuable. To identify resources is to learn what the problems are in the fullest sense, which resources are relevant, and where potential allies might be found. To organize complementary action is to learn which initiatives can reinforce one another.

In many ways, public learning is renaming, reframing, and deciding again—after the fact. It is deliberation in reverse. The questions are much the same: Should we have done what we did? Was it really consistent with what we now think is most important?

A learning community is like the ideal student who reads everything assigned and then goes to the library or surfs the Internet to find out more. This student does not copy a model or use a formula. Imitation is limitation. Learning communities study what others have done, but they adapt what they see to their own circumstances.

Learning communities also know how to fail successfully. Civic enterprises that aim for success tend to stop once goals have been met, even if problems remain. Likewise, projects that do not succeed disappoint people, and they too stop. So success and failure can have the same result: people quit in either case. But when communities are learning, they tend to push ahead because they look beyond success and failure. As Rudyard Kipling wrote, they "treat those two imposters just the same." If their work goes well, they try to improve on it. If they fail, they learn from their mistakes.

Six practices in one

> Attendance at the Suggsville association meetings continued to rise and fall, depending on which problems were being addressed. Some citizens dropped out because the association refused to get drawn into local election campaigns or to endorse special causes. Few worried about these fluctuations in participation because they considered it more important to build ties with other civic groups and rural neighborhood coalitions, as well as with institutions such as the county sheriff's office, economic development office, and health department. Creating networks around projects seemed more important than getting up to scale on any one project.
>
> Suggsville would not make anyone's list of model communities today; still, the town's citizens have increased their capacity to influence their own future. Asked what the civic initiatives produced, one Suggsvillian said, "When people banded together to make this a better place to live, it became a better place to live."[18]

The secret of democratic practices is that they are not stand-alone techniques; they fit inside one another like the wooden *matrëshka* nesting dolls from Russia. When people lay out their options for acting on a problem, they continue to mull over the name that best captures what is really at issue. Even as they move toward making a decision, they continue to revise both the framework and the name of the problem. As they deliberate, people anticipate what actions will have to be taken and what commitments they will have to make. They recall lessons learned from past efforts. Citizens may make commitments to act while they are still deliberating. The six practices are essential elements in the larger politics of people ruling themselves.

Practical Applications

What would it mean if public health practitioners thought of the public in a democratic rather than just a demographic sense? Practitioners themselves could surely answer that question better than anyone at the Kettering Foundation, which is not an authority on public health and is not in a position to write a prescription for aligning professional routines with democratic practices. The foundation is depending on public health practitioners to take up this challenge, and several opportunities to undertake alignment efforts have occurred.

Professionals who are aware of the importance of democratic practices usually want to know where to begin. Some have started by working with citizens to name issues in public terms; others have begun by encouraging deliberative decision making in forums. Where they start, however, seems less important than recognizing that these practices are just parts of a larger whole, of a democratic way of governing.

In their book on deliberative democracy, Gutmann and Thompson argue that democratic practices such as deliberation belong anywhere and everywhere—in civic organizations, in school boards, in tenants' associations.[19] There is no one right place to begin. However, beginning in a democratic fashion is essential if the objective is to strengthen democratic self-rule. Jay Rosen, a journalist who has worked with the Kettering Foundation, has stated the matter succinctly: the way someone enters politics has to be consistent with the politics they want to encourage. It is counterproductive to inaugurate a project of choice work with a citizenry that has not chosen to participate.

It is also unrealistic to try to stop a community in the midst of solving a problem and ask people to start over by renaming the issue at hand. Professionals would be better advised to look for opportunities in what is already taking place and to work on introducing democratic questions into the regular routines of naming, framing, and so on: Does anyone see another side to this problem? Are there other options we should consider? Almost everyone thinks we should do this, but are there any negative consequences we ought to examine? Rather than trying to teach deliberative decision making as a skill, it may be more effective to just start deliberating.

The Kettering Foundation has also seen experiments by health professionals to engage citizens who are engaging other citizens. They treat the public as more than a fixed or static body—an audience, a constituency, an electorate. There is a sense in which the public is not static at all; rather, it is a dynamic force, more like electricity than a lightbulb. Practices are in motion. This is why experiments in which professionals try to engage citizens engaging citizens are so important. To follow through on this analogy, these professionals are plugging into electricity rather than holding on to a lightbulb.

Scutchfield and his colleagues at the University of Kentucky College of Public Health have conducted such experiments in several communities using deliberative forums. They have reported a greater use of local resources to address problems and a greater sense of public ownership of problems. The public health practitioners they worked with also seem to have become more comfortable with public deliberation rather than relying on familiar routines such as commissioning studies or conducting focus group research.[20, 21]

Other pioneers using democratic concepts of the public include Laura Hall Downey at the University of Southern Mississippi, who argues that protecting the public's health requires dealing with problems that do not have clear-cut solutions. She suggests that practitioners look beyond their expertise to see whether useful insights can be found in the public arena.[22, 23] The University of Arkansas College of Public Health, working with a citizens' group called the Tri-County Rural Health Network, buys Downey's suggestion. What they learned from a series of community forums led to changes in the college's clinical programs—changes that eventually produced significant cost savings for the state's Medicaid program.[24]

And on another front, Sandral Hullett, working in rural Eutaw, Alabama, was the model for the Suggsville story about breast cancer.[17] She showed that deliberations on what to do about alarming rates of breast cancer could help increase screenings. Her work confirmed what Kurt Lewin had found earlier about the power of collective decision making to change behaviors.[25]

The foundation does not claim that any of these experiments were prompted merely by reflecting on a democratic understanding of the public, yet all of them mirror that understanding. That is, all the experiments treated citizens either as political actors with the potential to make sound policy decisions or as producers of public goods.

The experiments we have seen so far suggest that there is great promise in further experimentation. Already, textbooks and some courses deal with democratic values such as personal freedom. It would be only a short step to look at democratic practices, even if that requires delving into a new literature on citizens and communities.

Arguably, citizens and practitioners alike would benefit if the manner in which health care professionals and institutions went about their work were better aligned with the work citizens do. The two could reinforce each other at a time when the health care system is staggering under the burdens of escalating costs and a loss of public confidence in major institutions. But showing how this alignment can occur will require more public health practitioners who are willing to conduct experiments, which may occur more readily among new practitioners entering the field.

Notes

I am greatly indebted to Dr. Laura Hall Downey and my colleagues Dr. Alice Diebel and Melinda Gilmore for editing the manuscript for this chapter.

1. Woodruff P. *First Democracy: The Challenge of an Ancient Idea.* New York: Oxford University Press; 2005.

2. The Kettering Foundation developed its concept of *civic work* by drawing from the concept of *public work* in Boyte HC, Kari NN. *Building America: The Democratic Promise of Public Work.* Philadelphia: Temple University Press; 1996.

3. Schoch-Spana M, et al. Community engagement: Leadership tool for catastrophic health events. *Biosecurity and Bioterrorism: Biodefense Strategy Pract Sci.* 2007;5(1):8, 10–11.

4. Ostrom E. *Governing the Commons: The Evolution of Institutions for Collective Action.* New York: Cambridge University Press; 1990.

5. Milstein B. *Hygeia's Constellation: Navigating Health Futures in a Dynamic and Democratic World.* Atlanta: Centers for Disease Control and Prevention; April 15, 2008:54–57.

6. Project CLEAR: Community Leadership to Effect Air Emission Reductions (Final Report, June 2002). The public health official at the time was Michael Pompili—one of the most innovative public health officials I have encountered in my research.

7. See *Citizen Voices on Pandemic Flu Choices: A Report of the Public Engagement Pilot Project on Pandemic Influenza,* December 2005. The Keystone Center produced a subsequent report on this research: *The Public Engagement Project on Community Control Measures for Pandemic Influenza.* Keystone, CO: Keystone Center; May 2007.

8. McKnight J, Kretzmann J. *Building Communities from the Inside Out: A Path toward Finding and Mobilizing a Community's Assets.* Chicago: ACTA Publications; 1993. McKnight and Kretzmann show that even people in the most impoverished communities can generate their own power. These two scholars have documented what can happen when the collective abilities of people, not just their needs, are recognized.

9. The Suggsville story is drawn from more than fifty communities observed over thirty years. These include Tupelo, Mississippi, as described by Grisham VL. *Tupelo: The Evolution of a Community.* Dayton, OH: Kettering Foundation Press; 1999; and "Smalltown," Alabama, as described by Sumners JA, with Slaton C, Arthur J. *Building Community: The Uniontown Story.* Dayton, OH: Kettering Foundation; 2005. Also see

For Communities to Work. Dayton, OH: Kettering Foundation; 2002, and the description of Eutaw, Alabama, in Brown KA. Building a healthy community. *Kettering Rev.* 2005;23(1):42–51.

10. The practices presented here are based on insights about how democracy should work. Being normative, these insights are not like the findings of social scientists. However, the practices based on these insights are real—that is, they have all occurred at various times in many different places. The way the practices are described by Kettering reflects the foundation's conceptualization of experience.

11. Berry W. *The Unsettling of America: Culture and Agriculture.* San Francisco: Sierra Club Books; 1986:viii.

12. The practice of framing issues in this fashion has a thirty-year track record of countering polarization. The issue books of the National Issues Forums Institute have been used in thousands of public forums sponsored by a nonpartisan network of civic, educational, religious, and professional groups that promote nonpartisan public deliberation in communities around the country. To learn more, visit http://www.nifi.org.

13. In the "Funeral Oration of Pericles," Pericles describes public deliberation as *"prodidacthenai . . . logo,"* or the talk Athenians use to teach themselves before they act. See Thucydides, 2.40.2.

14. The concept of stages of deliberation comes from Yankelovich D. *Coming to Public Judgment: Making Democracy Work in a Complex World.* Syracuse, NY: Syracuse University Press; 1991.

15. For more information on covenants, see Elazar DJ, Kincaid J. Covenant and polity. *New Conversations.* 1979;4(Fall):4–8.

16. Stone CN. Linking civic capacity and human capital formation. In: Gittell MJ, ed. *Strategies for School Equity: Creating Productive Schools in a Just Society.* New Haven, CT: Yale University Press; 1998:163–176.

17. See Brown KA. Building a healthy community. *Kettering Rev.* 2005;23(1):42–51.

18. A similar comment was actually made by a citizen from the Naugatuck Valley community in Connecticut. See Brecher J. "If all the people are banded together": The Naugatuck Valley Project. In: Brecher J, Costello T, eds. *Building Bridges: The Emerging Grassroots Coalition of Labor and Community.* New York: Monthly Review Press; 1990:93.

19. Gutmann A, Thompson D. *Democracy and Disagreement.* Cambridge, MA: Belknap Press of Harvard University Press; 1996.

20. Scutchfield FD, Ireson C. *Kentucky Commonwealth Common Health Conversations for Health Action: A Review of Successful Communities.* Dayton, OH: Kettering Foundation; 2009.

21. Brown KA. *Community-Driven Health Initiatives in Kentucky Project Memoranda No. 2.* Dayton, OH: Kettering Foundation; July 30, 2006.

22. Scutchfield FD, Hall L, Ireson CL. The public and public health organizations: Issues for community engagement in public health. *Health Policy.* 2006;77:76–85.

23. Scutchfield FD, Ireson CL, Hall L. The voice of the public in public health policy and planning: The role of public judgment. *J Public Health Policy.* 2004;25(4):197–205.

24. For a report on the Arkansas project, see Felix HC, et al. *Linking Residents to*

Long-Term Care Services: First-Year Findings from the Community Connector Program Evaluation. Baltimore: Johns Hopkins University Press; 2007.

25. Lewin K. Group decision and social change. In: *Readings in Social Psychology.* New York: Henry Holt; 1952:459–473.

6

Public Health Services and Systems Research

Building the Science of Public Health Practice

Glen P. Mays, Paul K. Halverson, and William J. Riley

Despite spending far more resources on health care than any other nation on earth, the United States continues to lag behind many other industrialized nations in population health outcomes ranging from life expectancy at birth and infant mortality to the incidence of preventable chronic diseases.[1] Although many factors contribute to this gap between investment and outcome, one likely explanation is the limited resources and attention devoted to public health—that is, the activities designed to promote health and prevent disease and disability on a population-wide basis.[2-4] These activities include monitoring and reporting on community health status, investigating and controlling disease outbreaks, educating the public about health risks and prevention strategies, developing and enforcing laws and regulations to protect health, and inspecting and ensuring the safety and quality of water, food, air, and other resources necessary for health.[5] The vast majority of the $2.7 trillion spent on health in the United States each year supports the organization, financing, and delivery of medical care services, with less than 3 percent allocated to population-based public health strategies.[6,7] Meanwhile, the nation's health research enterprise focuses primarily on discovering new medical interventions and better ways of delivering these interventions to patients, with comparatively little attention given to uncovering new and better ways of preventing disease through public health.

A constellation of developments over the past decade calls attention to the need to strengthen the nation's public health system and its ability to protect its residents from preventable diseases and injuries. Both natural and man-made health threats have placed greater demands on the public health system, including new and resurgent infectious diseases such as SARS and pandemic influenza; the persistent risks of bioterrorism; such natural disasters as hurricanes and earthquakes, which may be occurring with increasing frequency and intensity due to climate change; evolving threats to food safety; and the rapid increase in obesity and preventable chronic diseases. In response, the federal government has invested more than $10 billion to support public health activities since 2001, with a primary focus on helping communities prepare for and deal with large-scale public health emergencies. More recently, the 2010 federal health reform legislation known as the Affordable Care Act (ACA) authorized the creation of a Prevention and Public Health Fund with $15 billion for public health activities over ten years.[8] At the same time, a global economic recession has caused governments at all levels to reduce funding for public health programs, forcing difficult decisions about which activities to support or scale back.

These changes highlight fundamental uncertainties about how best to invest in and deliver public health strategies to the populations that can obtain the most benefit from them. The nation's local, state, and federal public health agencies—together with their peers and partners in the private and public sectors—represent a vast yet diffuse delivery system charged to greater or lesser degrees with implementing these strategies.[9, 10] Unfortunately, evidence about the most effective and efficient ways of organizing, financing, and deploying public health strategies across this delivery system is extremely limited.[11, 12] Public health leaders have few research-tested guidelines, protocols, and decision supports to inform their choices with regard to funding, staffing, and managing public health activities. Similarly, policy leaders have relatively little empirical evidence to tell them how to use taxing, spending, and regulatory authorities most effectively in public health. This dearth of evidence promotes wide variation in public health practices across communities, raising the possibility of harmful, wasteful, and inequitable differences in practice.[13] The field of public health services and systems research (PHSSR) has grown rapidly in recent years to address these information needs and build the evidence required for improved decision making in public health practice. This chapter examines recent progress in the field of PHSSR and its application to contemporary issues in public health.

PHSSR and the Research Continuum

PHSSR exists within the larger continuum of health sciences research that seeks to discover innovations that improve human health (figure 6.1). At the left end of the continuum, *basic scientific research* uncovers the fundamental biomedical and environmental mechanisms that contribute to disease and disability processes. Moving through the continuum, *intervention research* uses the findings from basic science to develop and test the efficacy of health interventions in preventing, detecting, or treating disease and disability. At the right end of the continuum, *services and systems research* uses findings from intervention studies to design and test mechanisms for delivering efficacious interventions to populations that can benefit from them. These studies seek to answer a wide range of questions involving how best to deliver evidence-tested health interventions in real-world practice settings, including the following:

- What organizational, human, technological, and information resources are required to produce public health interventions, and how can the availability of these resources be assured?
- Who should pay for the delivery of public health interventions, using what types of financing mechanisms and payment methods?
- What factors influence the accessibility, reach, fidelity, quality, and cost of these interventions?
- What are the health and economic effects of the interventions when delivered in real-world settings?
- How and why do the effects of interventions vary across population subgroups and practice settings?

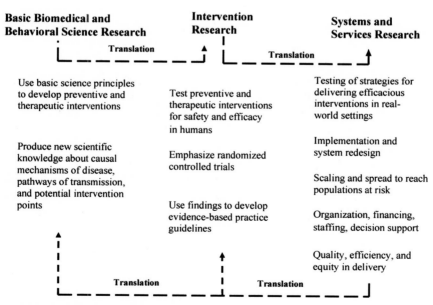

Figure 6.1. Health research continuum.

These studies produce the evidence needed to inform the decisions faced by health professionals, administrators, policy makers, and the public at large concerning how to deploy health resources in the most effective, efficient, and equitable ways possible.

The field of health services research plays a dominant role in the scientific pursuits listed on the right-hand side of this research continuum, although historically, health services research has focused narrowly on the delivery of medical care services, paying comparatively little attention to the delivery of public health interventions.[12] PHSSR fills this gap in the research continuum by supporting evaluative studies of the implementation and impact of public health strategies delivered on a population-wide basis, including public health laws and regulations, health information and education campaigns, disease surveillance and epidemiologic investigation, community health planning and mobilization efforts, and other initiatives designed to improve a population's health.

Placed in the context of other health-related research, PHSSR can be defined as "a field of inquiry that examines the organization, financing, and delivery of public health services at local, state, and national levels, and the impact of these services in population health."[14] The concept of public health services contained in this definition includes the full range of strategies to promote health and prevent disease on a population-wide basis. It is based on the Institute of Medicine's framework of three core public health functions: assessing population health needs and risks, developing and implementing policies to protect health, and assuring the delivery of effective interventions to maintain and improve health.[5]

Several defining elements of PHSSR distinguish this field from other scientific pursuits in health and health care. First, PHSSR studies are applied in nature and thereby seek to address questions, problems, and uncertainties related to the delivery of public health strategies faced by real-world public health decision makers.[13] Studies that seek to elucidate the fundamental determinants and mechanisms of health and disease are generally beyond the scope of PHSSR, as are studies that seek to establish the efficacy of specific public health interventions. Second, PHSSR studies investigate public health strategies as implemented in real-world public health settings, as opposed to ideal or highly controlled settings. The goal of these studies is to produce evidence about strategies that work in typical practice settings and with representative population groups encountered in public health practice. Third, PHSSR studies are practice based and seek to incorporate on-the-ground knowledge and experience acquired by public health professionals into their design and execution. This approach helps ensure that study findings will be relevant to and readily adopted in public health practice settings. Fourth, PHSSR studies go beyond estimating the "average" effects of public health strategies; they examine the extent to which strategies work better in some practice settings than in others and the extent to which strategies produce greater benefits for some population groups than for others. PHSSR studies therefore produce evidence about which strategies work best, in which institutional and community contexts, for which population groups, and why—a perspective that is also being used with increasing frequency in health care quality improvement research and other social program and policy research.[15-17]

Historical Foundations and Milestones

While research on public health delivery may appear to be a relatively new phenomenon, studies of this nature began at least as early as the beginning of the twentieth century.[18] During the 1910s, the American Medical Association took on the responsibility for assessing and comparing state public health agencies to ascertain their structures and operations and make recommendations for improving their services.[12] Responsibility for conducting these types of studies, and companion research that focused on local public health agencies, was subsequently assumed by the American Public Health Association and its Committee on Administrative Practices, which continued in some form into the 1950s. The culmination of this effort was Emerson's report on the organizational structures and human resources needed by local health departments to perform basic public health functions in six areas: communicable disease control, maternal and child health, vital statistics registration, public health laboratories, environmental health, and health education.[19] These early studies used research methods and data that left much to be desired, but their aim of producing evidence to inform policy and practice made them influential milestones along the path toward PHSSR.

Advances in public health research slowed during the 1960s through 1980s, when the nation's policy and research attention turned to medical care financing and cost containment through innovations such as Medicare, Medicaid, community health centers, and commercial HMOs. Several decades of inattention to public health programs and services led the National Academy of Sciences' Institute of Medicine (IOM) to release a landmark assessment of the nation's public health system in 1988, which concluded that the system was in disarray and in need of significant revitalization and restructuring.[5] Many of the public health research and practice initiatives launched in the years since that report's publication have been a direct response to its findings and recommendations. Among its many contributions, the report articulated a conceptual model of public health practice based on the three overarching responsibilities, or core functions, mentioned earlier. These were subsequently expanded into a set of ten essential services for public health by a federal working group that initially convened to define the role of public health in President Clinton's health reform agenda of the early 1990s.[20] These two conceptual frameworks underpin many of the contemporary research initiatives in public health delivery.

The IOM report stimulated a flurry of initiatives during the 1990s that were designed to measure and improve the delivery of public health services. At the beginning of the decade, the U.S. Department of Health and Human Services established its *Healthy People 2000* national health objectives—one of which was that by the year 2000, at least 90 percent of the population would be served by a public health department that effectively carried out the IOM core functions of assessment, policy development, and assurance.[21] In response, professional groups such as the National Association of County and City Health Officials (NACCHO) developed guidelines and self-assessment tools to help public health agencies translate and apply the IOM concepts to practice. NACCHO's Assessment Protocol for Excellence in Public Health (APEX/PH) and subsequent protocols were designed to guide agencies through the process of community health assessment. At the same time, the Centers for Disease Control and Prevention (CDC) commissioned a series of research projects to develop strategies to measure how well public health agencies performed the IOM core functions and related services. These projects are recognized as some of the earliest efforts to measure the performance of national samples of public health agencies in order to assess variation and change in public health practice.[18, 22-26] NACCHO also began to perform periodic surveys of the nation's local health departments, providing national data about the organization, operation, and staffing of local public health agencies.[27]

The acts of terrorism and bioterrorism that occurred in the United States in 2001 ushered in a period of heightened visibility for the public health system and allowed improvement efforts to transition from a diverse collection of small, independent projects to coordinated, large-scale initiatives. The CDC and several national public health associations launched the National Public Health Performance Standards Program (NPHPSP) in 2002 to develop consensus-based performance standards for state and local public health delivery systems, along with a process for collecting and comparing measures of compliance with these standards.[28] Designed as a voluntary self-assessment process, the NPHPSP focuses on the performance of public health systems—defined as the collective efforts of governmental and private organizations to deliver public health services for a defined community or state. Since its launch, hundreds of state and local public health systems have participated in the program, and the data collected have been used to support several important studies of performance variation.[29, 30]

At the same time, accreditation programs for public health agencies were created to serve as mechanisms to stimulate widespread involvement in performance measurement and improvement activities. Several states launched such accreditation programs during this period, including Michigan, Missouri, and North Carolina.[31] Many other states developed formal performance review and reporting initiatives designed to achieve similar objectives.[32] With support from the Robert Wood Johnson Foundation and the CDC, a voluntary national accreditation program for state and local public health agencies was launched in 2011, along with a research and evaluation infrastructure designed to monitor the effects of accreditation on public health delivery.[33]

Developmental Pathways for PHSSR

Like other fields of scientific inquiry, PHSSR builds evidence through cumulative developmental processes involving multiple studies conducted over time (figure 6.2). This process begins with *descriptive studies* designed to document important characteristics of public health delivery and to quantify the nature and extent of variation in public health practices and outcomes. For example, a descriptive study of food-borne illness prevention practices in a representative sample of communities might document how often food service establishments are inspected in each community, how often reports of suspected food-borne illnesses are investigated, and what protocols and methods are used to conduct these inspections and investigations. Next, *formative research studies* are often used to generate hypotheses about the mechanisms that give rise to variation in practices and outcomes. Often, qualitative research techniques are used to elicit the knowledge, experiences, and perceptions of key stakeholders who are involved in the practices or outcomes under study. In the food-borne illness example, focus groups and key informant interviews might be conducted with food service inspectors, food service workers, and customers of food service establishments in selected communities to examine stakeholder perceptions and experiences related to factors that influence the effectiveness of food safety inspections and outbreak investigations.

As a third step in the developmental process, *inferential studies* examine the causes and consequences of variation in public health practices. These studies explore cause-and-effect relationships among the factors that precipitate or contribute to practice variation. PHSSR is particularly interested in elucidating the effects of system characteristics, such as organizational structures

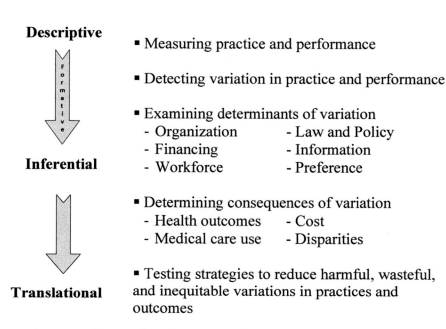

Descriptive

- Measuring practice and performance

- Detecting variation in practice and performance

- Examining determinants of variation
  - Organization   - Law and Policy
  - Financing   - Information
  - Workforce   - Preference

Inferential

- Determining consequences of variation
  - Health outcomes   - Cost
  - Medical care use   - Disparities

- Testing strategies to reduce harmful, wasteful, and inequitable variations in practices and outcomes

Translational

Figure 6.2. Developmental progression of public health services and systems research.

and interorganizational relationships, workforce characteristics and competencies, funding levels and financing mechanisms, information and communication resources, and community needs and preferences, in shaping patterns of practice variation. For example, a study might examine how the number of full-time equivalent sanitarians employed by a local health department and the number of licensed food vendors in the community influence the frequency or quality of the food service inspections performed. Importantly, inferential studies in PHSSR also seek to identify the health and economic consequences of practice variation in public health, relying heavily on quasi-experimental research designs and advanced statistical and econometric modeling techniques commonly used in outcomes research. In the food-borne illness example, such a study might test for evidence of higher case rates of food-borne illnesses and hospitalizations in communities that conduct less frequent food service inspections and case investigations and exhibit less fidelity to evidence-based protocols.

Collectively, inferential studies allow the PHSSR field to distinguish appropriate from unwarranted variation in public health delivery and to prioritize strategies for reducing unwarranted variation. Typically, variation in public health delivery is considered appropriate when it reflects differences in a population's needs, preferences, or values. For example, the volume and intensity of tobacco control activities delivered by the public health system in Salt Lake City are lower than those delivered in Philadelphia—which can be considered at least partially appropriate because smoking rates are lower in Salt Lake City than in Philadelphia. Tailoring public health strategies to the community's needs and preferences may yield more effective and efficient prevention efforts because resources can be targeted to the populations at greatest risk, and communities can be directly engaged in the design and implementation of public health strategies, enhancing community awareness, support, and compliance. Variation in public health delivery is considered unwarranted when it reflects the underuse of effective public health resources and practices (harmful variation), the overuse or unnecessary use of resources and practices (wasteful variation), or disparities in resources and practices that result in gaps in health protection for certain subgroups within the population (inequitable variation).[13]

A final step in the PHSSR developmental pathway is to use evidence from inferential studies to mount *translational studies* that develop and test strategies for improving public health delivery and reducing unwarranted variation in practice. These types of studies increasingly rely on modern quality improvement techniques borrowed from the field of industrial and systems engineering, such as root cause analysis, statistical process control, failure modes and effects analysis, and rapid-cycle learning collaborative.[34, 35] Translational studies may test the use of decision support tools, including practice guidelines and protocols, such as those in the CDC's *Guide to Community Preventive Services*; checklists and decision prompts; and performance measurement, reporting, and benchmarking tools. The PHSSR field is also keenly interested in translational studies that can evaluate the implementation and impact of the accreditation standards and performance measures that are being used with increasing frequency in the field of public health, including a new national voluntary accreditation program for state and local public health agencies.

Current State of the Field

In recent years, practice-based initiatives to improve public health delivery have far outpaced the development of rigorous research studies to inform and guide these initiatives. As a result, the methods currently used to measure performance and stimulate improvements stand on a relatively thin scientific base. The IOM acknowledged this problem in 2003 in a follow-up to its 1988 report on the public health system, noting in its preamble: "The Committee had hoped to provide specific guidance elaborating on the types and levels of workforce, infrastructure, related resources, and financial investments necessary to ensure the availability of essential public health services to all of the nation's communities. However, such evidence is limited, and there is no agenda or support for this type of research, despite the critical need for such data to promote and protect the nation's health."[36] Much of the existing research on public health services and delivery systems is descriptive in nature, providing an important base for future studies but offering little specific guidance to public health decision makers who want to improve practice. For example, recent studies provide a detailed view of how public health agencies are organized, what types of services they provide, and how these agencies are staffed and financed.[37-41] They highlight the extreme heterogeneity in organization and operation that exists across the nation's public health system. Data from 2005, for example, indicate that the smallest local public health agencies spend less than $1 per capita on their operations, while the largest agencies spend more than $200 per capita.[42] This heterogeneity complicates the task of conducting rigorous, comparative studies of public health practice. Nevertheless, recent work has demonstrated the feasibility of classifying public health agencies and delivery systems into relatively homogeneous groups for the purposes of analysis and comparison.

In a similar vein, researchers have used measures of performance from self-assessment instruments, such as the NPHPSP, to document wide variation in the range of activities performed by public health agencies and to explore the institutional and economic characteristics that account for some of this variation.[29, 30, 43] Although these types of studies offer important insight into the delivery of public health services, their utility and relevance are limited by the lack of any objective, validated methods of measuring the quality of public health practice in terms of effectiveness, timeliness, efficiency, and equity. Fortunately, advances in the fields of behavioral research and prevention research are leading to the discovery of an expanding collection of efficacious public health interventions. These can then be translated into evidence-based guidelines for public health practice, such as the U.S. Department of Health and Human Services' *Guide to Community Preventive Services*. These types of guidelines offer a starting point for creating process-based quality measures that reflect the extent to which public health agencies provide guideline-concordant services. Researchers have recently begun to explore methods of measuring how well public health practices conform to guidelines in the areas of emergency preparedness[44] and obesity prevention,[45-47] but further methodological advances are needed.

Policy and administrative decision makers are interested in understanding the health and economic impacts of investments in public health activities, but so far, relatively few studies have been able to isolate these effects reliably.[48] Conducting outcomes research on public health practice is complicated by the fact that many population health outcomes are determined by the cumulative impact of multiple factors over relatively long periods, making it difficult to isolate the contributions made by the actions of public health agencies. Heavy reliance on observational research designs and aggregated measures of population health makes these studies vulnerable to problems of selection bias, confounding, endogeneity, and ecological fallacy. Moreover, these studies often focus on outcomes that are relatively rare events—infectious disease outbreaks, natural disasters, or deaths from specific preventable causes. Achieving sufficient statistical power and precision to estimate the impact of public health actions on these types of outcomes can be challenging, particularly in small areas.

Research Example: Understanding the Organization of Public Health Delivery Systems

In the United States, public health services are delivered through the collective actions of governmental and private organizations that vary widely in their resources, missions, and operations. This complexity in interorganizational and intergovernmental structure has led to the widespread perception among policy makers and administrators that public health agencies defy meaningful description and comparison. Nevertheless, obtaining a better understanding of the organizational and operational attributes of public health delivery systems is a critical step in elucidating pathways for the improvement of public health services.

To facilitate the production of such evidence, researchers developed a new empirical method of classifying and comparing public health delivery systems, based on their organizational structure and functional characteristics.[10] This research used the IOM definition of a public health delivery system, which encompasses the full array of governmental and nongovernmental organizations that contribute to the delivery of essential public health services for a defined community or population. The typology focuses on delivery systems operating at the local level, but it can be extended to state-level systems. Related typologies developed in the health services research literature have proved extremely valuable for policy and administrative decision making, as well as for ongoing research. For example, the typologies of hospital networks and systems developed by Shortell, Bazzoli, and colleagues over the past two decades have served in numerous policy and administrative applications concerning the regulation, coordination, and improvement of hospital-based health care services.[49, 50]

A typology of public health systems can enhance policy and administrative decision making as well as public health research. A typology allows "apples to apples" comparisons across communities to determine how public health services are organized and delivered. Such comparisons can form the basis of public health performance assessment activities and inform the development of performance standards for public health agencies, such as those being used as part of state and national accreditation programs for public health agencies.

To develop the typology, researchers collected data through a national longitudinal survey of local public health agencies serving communities with at least 100,000 residents. The survey measured the availability of twenty core public health activities in local communities and the types of organizations contributing to each activity. In each community, the collection of organizations that contributed to public health activities was defined as the *local public health delivery system*. Cluster analysis was used to group these local public health delivery systems, based on observed similarities in three characteristics: (1) the scope of activities delivered in the community, (2) the range of organizations contributing to these activities, and (3) the division of effort within the system, as indicated by the proportion of the total community effort to perform public health activities contributed by the local governmental public health agency. Data were collected first in 1998 and again in 2006 in order to examine changes in the structure of delivery systems over time.

Results of the study identified seven public health system configurations that can be grouped into three tiers, based on the scope of public health activities performed (differentiation). Three of the seven system configurations were identified as highly differentiated, meaning that they offered a broad and encompassing scope of activities. These systems generally performed more than two-thirds of the activities in each of the three IOM domains of assessment, policy development, and assurance. As such, these systems were labeled "comprehensive" in their scope of activities. Another two system configurations were identified as moderately differentiated because they performed about half the activities in each IOM domain. These systems were labeled "conventional" in differentiation because they aligned closely with the scope of services performed in the study's median community. The final two system configurations performed a relatively narrow scope of activities and were therefore labeled "limited" in differentiation. Public health systems frequently migrate from one configuration to another over time, with an overall trend toward offering a broader scope of services and engaging a wider range of organizations. The prevalence and attributes of each system configuration are summarized in table 6.1.

Table 6.1. Summary of the Seven Local Public Health System Configurations

Type of System and Prevalence	Description
Tier I: Comprehensive	
1. Concentrated comprehensive 1998: 12.5% 2006: 21.4%	• Broad scope of activities performed • Wide range of organizations participating in activities • Local public health agency shoulders much of the effort in performing activities
2. Distributed comprehensive 1998: 5.1% 2006: 3.9%	• Broad scope of activities performed • Wide range of organizations participating in activities • Effort in performing activities is distributed across participating organizations
3. Independent comprehensive 1998: 6.6% 2006: 11.6%	• Broad scope of activites performed • Narrow range of organizations participating in activities • Local public health agency shoulders much of the effort in performing activities
Tier II. Conventional	
4. Concentrated conventional (transitory system) 1998: 3.4% 2006: 3.0%	• Moderate scope of activities performed • Moderate range of organizations participating in activities • Local public health agency shoulders much of the effort in performing activities • Highly transitory system
5. Distributed conventional (modal system) 1998: 46.7% 2006: 30.9%	• Moderate scope of activities performed • Moderate range of organizations participating in activities • Effort in performing activities is distributed across participating organizations
Tier III. Limited	
6. Concentrated limited 1998: 12.3% 2006: 18.0%	• Narrow scope of activities performed • Limited range of organizations participating in activities • Local public health agency shoulders much of the effort in performing activities
7. Distributed limited 1998: 13.4% 2006: 11.2%	• Narrow scope of activities performed • Moderate range of organizations participating in activities • Effort in performing activities is distributed across participating organizations

Source: Data from Mays GP, Scutchfield FD, Bhandari MW, Smith SA. Understanding the organization of public health delivery systems: An empirical typology. *Milbank Q.* 2010;88(1):81–111.

Which system configurations work best in delivering public health activities? The answer is likely to depend in part on the institutional, political, and community context, but the public health system typology provides an empirical framework for examining this question systematically. By studying communities that change from one system configuration to another, it is possible to investigate how measures of public health performance and outcomes change in response, using statistical and econometric methods to control for general temporal trends and other confounding factors that influence performance and outcomes over time. This type of study, known as a difference-in-difference analysis, revealed that systems moving to one of the three comprehensive configurations over the 1998–2006 period showed the largest gains in the perceived effectiveness of public health activities, as reported by local public health officials in these communities (figure 6.3). These comprehensive systems also showed larger reductions in preventable mortality in the communities they served, compared with systems that moved to conventional or limited configurations. Surprisingly, the systems with the largest deficits in performance and outcomes were not those that moved to limited

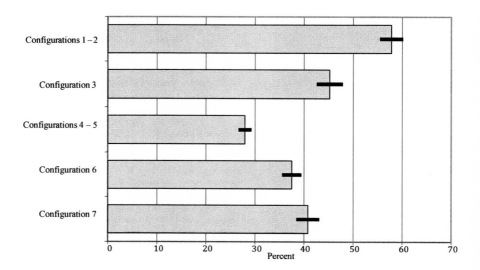

Figure 6.3. Differences in self-rated public health effectiveness across seven configurations of public health systems. *Note:* Horizontal lines indicate 95 percent confidence intervals for the estimates shown in the bar graphs. *Source:* Data from Mays GP, Scutchfield FD, Bhandari MW, Smith SA. Understanding the organization of public health delivery systems: An empirical typology. *Milbank Q.* 2010;88(1):81–111.

configurations; rather, the systems that moved to one of the two conventional configurations had the largest deficits. One possible explanation is that conventional systems may support too many public health activities with too few organizational partners and resources, resulting in lower overall effectiveness. By comparison, limited systems may focus their limited resources on a smaller scope of high-priority activities. Clearly, much more research is needed to elucidate structural and organizational mechanisms that can be used to improve public health system performance. The typology developed through this analysis can facilitate comparative studies to identify which delivery system configurations perform best in which contexts.

Research Example: Understanding Variation in Public Health Spending

Geographic variation in medical care spending has long been a source of policy concern because it implies large inefficiencies and inequities in resource use and availability. Recent PHSSR studies show that geographic variation in public health spending may be of even greater concern.[51-53] As policy makers struggle with how to reform the health care delivery system and how to pay for it, investments in public health and prevention should be part of the discussion, and sound empirical research on public health spending is needed to inform these policy decisions. Many of the costly chronic diseases that Americans suffer from can be prevented or delayed. If communities spend more on prevention, will they need to spend less on medical care to treat patients? If communities are spending more on medical care, does this mean they are not spending enough to keep people from getting sick in the first place? These are the tough questions policy makers face as they work to decide how to improve the health care system for all Americans.

To inform these issues, researchers used a longitudinal cohort design to analyze changes in public health spending patterns and population health measures among the nation's 3,000 local public health agencies over the twelve-year period 1993–2005. The NACCHO collected data on the organizational and financial characteristics of these agencies through census surveys fielded in 1989, 1993, 1997, 2005, and 2008. These data were linked with contemporaneous information on community characteristics, federal and state spending, cause-specific mortality rates, and area medical spending estimates from the Dartmouth Atlas of Health Care. Multivariate regression models were used to estimate how changes in public health spending influenced mortality from preventable causes and medical care spending levels, using instrumental-variables techniques to control for unmeasured factors that jointly influence spending and mortality.[54] This analysis produced a number of important findings:

- Wide geographic variation exists in public health spending across communities. When communities were grouped into quintiles based on their level of per capita public health spending, the top 20 percent of communities spent thirteen times more resources on public health activities than did the lowest 20 percent of communities.
- More than one-third of communities experienced reductions in per capita public health spending over the twelve-year period. Rural communities and communities with higher proportions of nonwhite residents were somewhat more likely to experience spending reductions.
- Communities with larger growth in public health spending experienced larger reductions in mortality from the leading preventable causes of death. After controlling for other factors, mortality rates fell by 1.2 percent to 6.9 percent for each 10 percent increase in public health spending, with the largest effects observed for infant mortality and deaths due to heart disease, diabetes, and cancer (figure 6.4).
- Communities with larger growth in public health spending experienced slower growth in the rate of medical care spending per person, as estimated using Medicare spending data. Each 10 percent increase in public health spending per capita was associated with a 5.7 percent reduction in the rate of growth in medical care spending per person.

Several factors may explain this relationship:

- Prevention: Availability and access to public health resources, such as preventive services, may offset the need for medical care in some communities by preventing or limiting the onset of disease and injury.
- Care substitution: In communities where rates of health insurance coverage are low and access to private medical providers is limited, more people may take advantage of the preventive and limited clinical services offered by public health agencies.
- Crowd-out: Communities that spend heavily on medical care may have fewer local resources available to invest in public health activities.

These research findings suggest that increasing public health investments in communities with historically low levels of spending may be an effective way of constraining medical costs and reducing geographic disparities in health. Findings have been used by policy analysts and public health officials

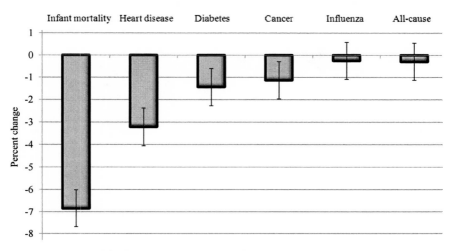

Figure 6.4. Estimated effects of a 10 percent increase in local public health spending on selected measures of preventable mortality, 1993–2005. *Note:* Vertical lines represent 95 percent confidence intervals for the estimates shown in the bar graphs. *Source:* Data from Mays GP, Smith SA. Evidence links increases in public health spending to declines in preventable deaths. *Health Aff.* 2011;30(8):1585–1593.

at the state and national levels to inform decisions on investments in public health infrastructure. For example, states have used the findings to decide how best to respond to state budget shortfalls precipitated by the economic downturn, helping to insulate the most vital public health activities from the largest funding cuts. At the federal level, these findings have been used to inform the design and implementation of the Prevention and Public Health Fund authorized by the ACA.

Strengthening the Science Base through Practice-Based Research

A weakness of many existing PHSSR activities has been public health practitioners' lack of direct engagement in the design and conduct of this research, resulting in relatively low levels of research awareness and research use among them. Practitioners often cannot see how research findings can be used to improve everyday public health decision making, and researchers often fail to identify clear practice implications and feasible improvement strategies that flow from their scholarship. To address these issues, researchers are beginning to use the concept of a practice-based research network (PBRN), with the goals of using practitioner input to develop and implement

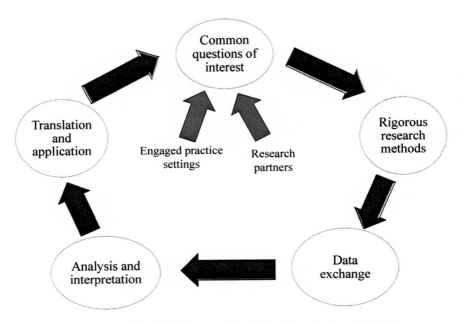

Figure 6.5. Conceptual model for a public health practice-based research network.

new PHSSR studies and accelerating the translation of research findings into new policies and practice strategies that improve health. A PBRN brings multiple public health agencies and research partners together to design and implement studies of population-based strategies that prevent disease and injury and promote health. Participating practitioners and researchers collaborate to identify questions of interest, design rigorous and relevant studies, execute feasible research effectively, and translate findings rapidly into practice (figure 6.5). As such, PBRNs can expand the volume and quality of practice-based research needed for evidence-based decision making in public health.

PBRNs have been used successfully in the field of health services research to study clinical innovations and test quality improvement strategies in community-based medical practice settings, largely with the engagement of practicing physicians and occasionally other health professionals.[55-57] Building on this model, the Robert Wood Johnson Foundation launched the Public Health PBRN Program in 2008.[58] Like their counterparts in clinical research, public health PBRNs are particularly well positioned to test and evaluate strategies for accelerating the diffusion of evidence-based practices and policies across a variety of practice settings. The range of public health studies that can be conducted through PBRNs is wide and includes the following:

- Comparative case studies designed to identify problems or innovations in how public health activities are currently implemented in different practice settings.
- Large-scale observational studies designed to evaluate practice variation across local or state public health settings to identify opportunities to reduce unnecessary, inefficient, or harmful variation.
- Intervention studies and community trials designed to test the effectiveness and cost-effectiveness of new public health programs. Such studies may also test the effectiveness of quality improvement initiatives directed at existing programs.
- Policy evaluations and natural experiments designed to monitor the effects of key policy and administrative changes made at the state or local level, such as changes in laws and regulations, shifts in funding or staffing levels, and organizational restructuring, such as service consolidation, regionalization, or decentralization.

These types of studies require the ability to measure public health activities and outcomes in real-world practice settings and to make valid comparisons across such settings and over time.

The Public Health PBRN Program currently supports twelve research networks comprising local and state governmental public health agencies, community partners, and collaborating academic research institutions. These networks are located in Colorado, Connecticut, Florida, Kentucky, Massachusetts, Minnesota, Nebraska, New York, North Carolina, Ohio, Washington, and Wisconsin. In addition to these twelve, other public health PBRNs participate as affiliate members and as emerging networks under development. The National Coordinating Center for the Public Health PBRN Program, located at the University of Kentucky, provides resources and technical assistance for the development and conduct of research projects. The center also organizes crosscutting and multinetwork research studies designed to evaluate and compare public health strategies implemented across diverse practice settings.

Research projects currently under way address a wide range of topics and delivery system issues. In the most general sense, all these projects focus on elucidating the causes or consequences of variation in the organization, financing, and delivery of public health services across communities. As such, the projects are designed to produce findings that will lead to a reduction in unwarranted variation and an improvement in the effectiveness, efficiency, and equity of public health practice. Issues to be addressed by the participating public health PBRNs include the following:

- Variation in staffing levels among local public health agencies and the impact on the volume and quality of public health services delivered.
- Variation in the implementation and impact of regionalized public health delivery models that consolidate the operations of multiple small agencies to achieve economies of scope and scale.
- Variation in local health department approaches to communicable disease reporting, and its impact on surveillance and disease control efforts.
- Impact of a comprehensive state public health reform law on the organization and delivery of local public health services.
- Causes and consequences of variation in the local public health response to the H1N1 influenza outbreak.
- Impact of recession-driven funding reductions on the delivery of evidence-based public health programs and services.
- Effectiveness of quality improvement strategies for diabetes prevention delivered through local public health agencies.
- Effectiveness of public health agencies' efforts to facilitate the adoption of evidence-based obesity prevention strategies by local community coalitions.

Although still relatively new, public health PBRNs show considerable promise in strengthening both the rigor and the relevance of PHSSR studies.

Next Steps and Future Directions

A number of other federal, state, and foundation-supported initiatives are now under way to expand the quantity and quality of research on public health services and systems. At the national level, the Robert Wood Johnson Foundation and the CDC have convened groups of researchers, public health officials, and other stakeholders to stimulate thinking on new avenues of inquiry, develop a consensus-based research agenda, and set research priorities to guide future studies. This broad-based agenda will complement and enhance earlier research agendas, including those devoted to public health systems,[59] public health workforce issues,[60] public health finance and economics,[48] public health preparedness,[61] and rural public health practice.[62]

Efforts are also under way to expand the limited funding available for studies of public health services and delivery systems—a situation that has long constrained the development of this field of inquiry. The CDC's Public

Health Practice Program Office periodically secured modest levels of funding for this type of research during the 1990s and early 2000s, but there was no stable and ongoing source of support, and the demise of this office during the CDC's 2004 reorganization placed continued federal funding in question. Since that time, the Robert Wood Johnson Foundation has made a significant commitment to this field by establishing competitive research grant programs in PHSSR; these programs are now directed through the National Coordinating Center for PHSSR at the University of Kentucky. The federal government has also stepped up investments in this area through the creation of a network of university-based centers for public health systems research related to emergency preparedness, authorized by the Pandemic and All-Hazards Preparedness Act of 2006.[61] Most recently, the 2010 ACA authorized a new federal program of research devoted to improving public health service delivery. These initiatives, working in tandem with the federal government's growing emphasis on translational research at the National Institutes of Health and other science agencies, promise to foster continued advances in PHSSR.

Efforts are ongoing to build and enhance core data resources on key elements of the public health delivery system, but more work is needed. Although longitudinal data sources exist to support the study of hospitals, physicians, health insurers, and other elements of the medical care system, there are no similar data sources for the organizations and workforces that deliver public health services. To address this issue, the Robert Wood Johnson Foundation recently funded a project to collect longitudinal data through periodic surveys of the nation's local public health agencies, state health agencies, and local boards of health. These new data sources will extend and expand on the data collected in the past by NACCHO. Researchers have begun to "harmonize" the data collected through these surveys, thereby ensuring that comparable data on organization, staffing, financing, and service delivery are collected at multiple levels of the public health system. Although these foundation-supported efforts to build data infrastructure for PHSSR are notable, contributions from the federal health data enterprise are needed as well.

Enhancing Translation and Impact

The field of PHSSR has the potential to fill an important gap in the nation's efforts to translate and apply biomedical and behavioral research to the solution of human health problems. Translational research has become a touchstone of the National Institutes of Health and other federal research agencies as they attempt to realize a greater health impact from the nation's investment in scientific research. However, current initiatives to strengthen translation have focused primarily on the "bench-to-bedside" issues involved in taking findings from research settings and moving them into routine patient care settings, such as hospitals and physician practices. There has been relatively little emphasis on engaging community and public health settings in these processes of knowledge transfer. Public health agencies are becoming increasingly important links in the chain of research translation, particularly for the growing body of biomedical and behavioral discoveries related to disease prevention and health promotion. As such, the field of PHSSR is ideally positioned to produce studies that can shed light on how best to incorporate new biomedical and behavioral discoveries into routine public health practice.

The current policy discourse around health reform reflects the need to emphasize prevention as part of the way to achieve a higher-performing health system. This goal will require more and better information about how to deliver effective prevention strategies to the populations that can most benefit from them. Although the field is still relatively new, PHSSR promises to contribute this type of information. As this field produces more and stronger evidence, policy makers and practitioners will increasingly look to these studies for guidance when making decisions to protect and promote health at the population level. The result, we hope, will be the public health system moving in tandem with the medical care system toward greater impact, value, equity, and accountability.

Notes

1. Davis K. *Health and Wealth: Measuring Health System Performance, Invited Testimony at the Hearing on Rethinking the Gross Domestic Product as a Measurement of National Strength.* Washington, DC: U.S. Senate Committee on Commerce, Science, and Transportation, Subcommittee on Interstate Commerce, Trade, and Tourism; 2008.

2. Lantz PM, Lichtenstein RL, Pollack HA. Health policy approaches to population health: The limits of medicalization. *Health Aff.* 2007;26(5):1253–1257.

3. Lee P, Paxman D. Reinventing public health. *Annu Rev Public Health.* 1997;18:1–35.

4. McGinnis MJ, Williams-Russo P, Knickman JR. The case for more active policy attention to health promotion. *Health Aff.* 2002;21:78–93.

5. Institute of Medicine. *The Future of Public Health.* Washington, DC: National Academies Press; 1988.

6. Brown R, Elixhauser A, Corea J, Luce B, Sheingold S. *National Expenditures for Health Promotion and Disease Prevention Activities in the United States.* Washington, DC: Batelle Medical Technology Assessment and Policy Research Center; 1991.

7. Sensenig AL. Refining estimates of public health spending as measured in the

National Health Expenditures Accounts: The U.S. experience. *J Public Health Manage Pract.* 2007;13(2):103–114.

8. Trust for America's Health. *Ready or Not? Protecting the Public's Health from Diseases, Disasters, and Bioterrorism.* Washington, DC: Trust for America's Health; 2010.

9. Mays GP, Scutchfield FD. Improving public health system performance through multiorganizational partnerships. *Prev Chronic Dis.* 2010;7(6):A116.

10. Mays GP, Scutchfield FD, Bhandari MW, Smith SA. Understanding the organization of public health delivery systems: An empirical typology. *Milbank Q.* 2010;88(1):81–111.

11. Scutchfield FD, Marks JS, Perez DJ, Mays GP. Public health services and systems research. *Am J Prev Med.* 2007;33(2):169–171.

12. Scutchfield FD, Mays GP, Lurie N. Applying health services research to public health practice: An emerging priority. *Health Serv Res.* 2009;44(5 Pt 2):1775–1787.

13. Mays GP, Smith SA, Ingram RC, Racster LJ, Lamberth CD, Lovely ES. Public health delivery systems: Evidence, uncertainty, and emerging research needs. *Am J Prev Med.* 2009;36(3):256–265.

14. Mays GP, Halverson PK, Scutchfield FD. Behind the curve? What we know and need to learn from public health systems research. *J Public Health Manage Pract.* 2003;9(3):179–182.

15. Pawson R, Tilley N. *Realistic Evaluation.* London; Thousand Oaks, CA: Sage; 1997.

16. Clancy CM, Berwick DM. The science of safety improvement: Learning while doing. *Ann Intern Med.* 2011;154(10):699–701.

17. Berwick DM. The science of improvement. *JAMA.* 2008;299(10):1182–1184.

18. Turnock BJ, Handler AS. From measuring to improving public health practice. *Annu Rev Public Health.* 1997;18:261–282.

19. American Public Health Association, Committee on Administrative Practice, Subcommittee on Local Health Units; Emerson H; Luginbulh M; Commonwealth Fund. *Local Health Units for the Nation.* New York: Commonwealth Fund; 1945.

20. Baker EL, Melton RJ, Stange PV, et al. Health reform and the health of the public: Forging community health partnerships. *JAMA.*1994;272(16):1276–1282.

21. U.S. Public Health Service. *Healthy People 2000: National Health Promotion and Disease Prevention Objectives: Full Report, with Commentary.* Washington, DC: U.S. Department of Health and Human Services; 1991.

22. Miller CA, Halverson P, Mays G. Flexibility in measurement of public health performance. *J Public Health Manage Pract.* 1997;3(5):vii–viii.

23. Miller CA, Moore KS, Richards TB, Monk JD. A proposed method for assessing the performance of local public health functions and practices. *Am J Public Health.* 1994;84(11):1743–1749.

24. Turnock BJ, Handler A, Hall W, Potsic S, Nalluri R, Vaughn EH. Local health department effectiveness in addressing the core functions of public health. *Public Health Rep.* 1994;109(5):653–658.

25. Turnock BJ, Handler AS, Hall W, Potsic S, Munson J, Vaughn EH. Roles for

state-level local health liaison officials in local public health surveillance and capacity building. *Am J Prev Med.* 1995;11(6 Suppl):41–44.

26. Turnock BJ, Handler AS, Miller CA. Core function-related local public health practice effectiveness. *J Public Health Manage Pract.* 1998;4(5):26–32.

27. Gerzoff RB, Gordon RL, Richards TB. Recent changes in local health department spending. *J Public Health Policy.* 1996;17(2):170–180.

28. Corso LC, Wiesner PJ, Halverson PK, Brown CK. Using the essential services as a foundation for performance measurement and assessment of local public health systems. *J Public Health Manage Pract.* 2000;6(5):1–18.

29. Mays GP, McHugh MC, Shim K, et al. Institutional and economic determinants of public health system performance. *Am J Public Health.* 2006;96(3):523–531.

30. Scutchfield FD, Knight EA, Kelly AV, Bhandari MW, Vasilescu IP. Local public health agency capacity and its relationship to public health system performance. *J Public Health Manage Pract.* 2004;10(3):204–215.

31. Beitsch LM, Thielen L, Mays G, et al. The multistate learning collaborative: States as laboratories: Informing the national public health accreditation dialogue. *J Public Health Manage Pract.* 2006;12(3):217–231.

32. Mays G, Beitsch LM, Corso L, Chang C, Brewer R. States gathering momentum: Promising strategies for accreditation and assessment activities in multistate learning collaborative applicant states. *J Public Health Manage Pract.* 2007;13(4):364–373.

33. Corso LC, Landrum LB, Lenaway D, Brooks R, Halverson PK. Building a bridge to accreditation—the role of the National Public Health Performance Standards Program. *J Public Health Manage Pract.* 2007;13(4):374–377.

34. Riley W, Brewer R. Review and analysis of quality improvement techniques in police departments: Application for public health. *J Public Health Manage Pract.* 2009;15(2):139–149.

35. Riley W, Parsons H, McCoy K, et al. Introducing quality improvement methods into local public health departments: Structured evaluation of a statewide pilot project. *Health Serv Res.* 2009;44(5 Pt 2):1863–1879.

36. Institute of Medicine, Committee on Assuring the Health of the Public in the 21st Century. *The Future of the Public's Health in the 21st Century.* Washington, DC: National Academies Press; 2003.

37. Madamala K, Sellers K, Beitsch LM, Pearsol J, Jarris PE. Structure and functions of state public health agencies in 2007. *Am J Public Health.* 2011;101(7):1179–1186.

38. Beitsch LM, Grigg M, Menachemi N, Brooks RG. Roles of local public health agencies within the state public health system. *J Public Health Manage Pract.* 2006;12(3):232–241.

39. Beitsch LM, Brooks RG, Grigg M, Menachemi N. Structure and functions of state public health agencies. *Am J Public Health.* 2006;96(1):167–172.

40. Tilson H, Gebbie KM. The public health workforce. *Annu Rev Public Health.* 2004;25:341–356.

41. Gebbie K, Merrill J, Tilson HH. The public health workforce. *Health Aff.* 2002;21(6):57–67.

42. National Association of County and City Health Officials. *2005 National Profile of Local Health Departments.* Washington, DC: NACCHO; 2006.

43. Mays GP, Halverson PK, Baker EL, Stevens R, Vann JJ. Availability and perceived effectiveness of public health activities in the nation's most populous communities. *Am J Public Health.* 2004;94(6):1019–1026.

44. Lurie N, Wasserman J, Stoto M, et al. Local variation in public health preparedness: Lessons from California. *Health Aff.* January–June 2004(Suppl Web ExclusivesW4):341–353.

45. Dodson EA, Baker EA, Brownson RC. Use of evidence-based interventions in state health departments: A qualitative assessment of barriers and solutions. *J Public Health Manage Pract.* 2010;16(6):E9–E15.

46. Brownson RC, Ballew P, Dieffenderfer B, et al. Evidence-based interventions to promote physical activity: What contributes to dissemination by state health departments. *Am J Prev Med.* 2007;33(1 Suppl):S66–S73; quiz S74–S68.

47. Slater SJ, Powell LM, Chaloupka FJ. Missed opportunities: Local health departments as providers of obesity prevention programs for adolescents. *Am J Prev Med.* 2007;33(4 Suppl):S246–S250.

48. Carande-Kulis VG, Getzen TE, Thacker SB. Public goods and externalities: A research agenda for public health economics. *J Public Health Manage Pract.* 2007;13(2):227–232.

49. Dubbs NL, Bazzoli GJ, Shortell SM, Kralovec PD. Reexamining organizational configurations: An update, validation, and expansion of the taxonomy of health networks and systems. *Health Serv Res.* 2004;39(1):207–220.

50. Bazzoli GJ, Shortell SM, Dubbs N, Chan C, Kralovec P. A taxonomy of health networks and systems: Bringing order out of chaos. *Health Serv Res.*1999;33(6):1683–1717.

51. Mays GP, Smith SA. Geographic variation in public health spending: Correlates and consequences. *Health Serv Res.* 2009;44(5 Pt 2):1796–1817.

52. Mays GP, Smith SA. Evidence links increases in public health spending to declines in preventable deaths. *Health Aff.* 2011;30(8):1585–1593.

53. Mays GP, McHugh MC, Shim K, et al. Getting what you pay for: Public health spending and the performance of essential public health services. *J Public Health Manage Pract.* 2004;10(5):435–443.

54. Newhouse JP, McClellan M. Econometrics in outcomes research: The use of instrumental variables. *Annu Rev Public Health.* 1998;19:17–34.

55. Kottke TE, Solberg LI, Nelson AF, et al. Optimizing practice through research: A new perspective to solve an old problem. *Ann Fam Med.* 2008;6(5):459–462.

56. Thomas P, Griffiths F, Kai J, O'Dwyer A. Networks for research in primary health care. *BMJ.* 2001;322(7286):588–590.

57. Fraser I, Lanier D, Hellinger F, Eisenberg JM. Putting practice into research. *Health Serv Res.* 2002;37(1):xiii–xxvi.

58. Mays GP. Leading improvement through inquiry: Practice-based research networks in public health. *Leadership in Public Health.* 2011;9(1):1–3.

59. Lenaway D, Halverson P, Sotnikov S, Tilson H, Corso L, Millington W. Public health systems research: Setting a national agenda. *Am J Public Health.* 2006;96(3):410–413.

60. Cioffi JP, Lichtveld MY, Tilson H. A research agenda for public health workforce development. *J Public Health Manage Pract.* 2004;10(3):186–192.

61. Institute of Medicine. *Research Priorities in Emergency Preparedness and Response for Public Health Systems: Letter Report.* Washington, DC: National Academies Press; 2008.

62. Meit M. Development of a rural public health research agenda. *Public Health Rep.* 2004;119(5):515–517.

7

National Accreditation of Public Health Departments

Kaye Bender

In September 2011 the first national public health department accreditation program opened its doors for business. The Public Health Accreditation Board (PHAB), chartered in May 2007, officially accomplished something first suggested in 1850. That year, *Report of the Sanitary Commission of Massachusetts* (the Shattuck Report) described an early framework of the determinants of health and set forth the duties of councils of health in assessing the public's health status and promoting interventions aimed at improving it.[1] In essence, these were early standards of public health and a call to action for implementation.

In 1914 the *Journal of the American Medical Association* (*JAMA*) published several articles that called on public health agencies to support standardization, efficiency, and a planned approach to delivering public health services.[2] Joseph Mountin, founder of the Centers for Disease Control and Prevention (CDC), described the importance of local health departments in carrying out governmental public health activities in an organized manner. A December 1945 paper entitled "A Twenty-five Year Review of the Work of the Committee on Administrative Practice" advocated regular reviews and reports on the performance of public health agencies, which "might be set up as a norm or as a general guide to be used by any community which aspires to provide adequate health protection for its citizens."[3]

For the next several decades, most of the literature describing the work of health departments was based on profile and observation, with no real attention given to performance measurement.[4] In 1988 the Institute of Medicine (IOM) report *The Future of Public Health* described the importance of a governmental presence in local communities, but it characterized the public health infrastructure as being in disarray.[5] Almost fifteen years later, another IOM report entitled *The Future of the Public's Health in the 21st Century* repeated that observation, citing the need for a public health "backbone" in every community—the local public health department.[6] That same study noted the important work initiated by the National Public Health Performance Standards Program (NPHPSP) in tracking trends in public health practice at the systems level, providing accountability to stakeholders and constituencies, benchmarking performance for improvement efforts, and increasing the scientific basis for public health practice. A recommendation for a national dialogue on the accreditation of public health departments was included in the 2003 IOM report.

The Robert Wood Johnson Foundation and the CDC cofunded a feasibility study on accreditation in 2005. The study was conducted by a twenty-five-member steering committee composed of representatives from public health departments, academia, and advocacy organizations. Two questions guided the study: Is it desirable to develop a national, voluntary public health accreditation program for the country? Is it feasible to initiate such a program? A report was issued in 2006, not only responding affirmatively to these questions but also suggesting a model for the development of national public health accreditation.[7] Simultaneous with this study, the Robert Wood Johnson Foundation funded another initiative, the Multistate Learning Collaborative (MLC); its aim was to both foster interest in accreditation and institute a culture of quality improvement in public health.[8] The Public Health Accreditation Board (PHAB) grew out of this study and was supported by the work of the MLC.

Although accreditation is not a new concept to many governmental businesses (e.g., public education, hospitals and health systems, fire departments, police departments), it is a new concept to public health. After many decades spent identifying the need and almost two decades of definitive preparatory work, PHAB's creation constitutes a historic moment in public health. The goal of PHAB's accreditation activities is to improve the performance and quality of state, local, tribal, and territorial public health departments in order to impact the health outcomes of the communities they serve.

It is important to recognize the difference between standards and accreditation. *Standards* can be defined as qualitative statements that reflect research-based best practices for a health department and function as the minimum requirements to achieve accreditation. *Accreditation* is the process by which an identified set of standards is utilized to evaluate an organization's performance and determine whether those standards have been met.

Development of the Public Health Accreditation Board

The initial recommendations from the 2006 Exploring Accreditation Project Report were realized when the Public Health Accreditation Board was incorporated and charged with administering the accreditation of national public health departments. From 2007 to 2011, PHAB developed its Board of Directors, recruiting state, local, and tribal public health leaders as members. Building on the successes of several state-based accreditation programs and the NPHPSP, a set of standards and measures was created and tested in both alpha and beta tests.

Thirty health departments that varied in size, organizational structure, scope of service delivery, and governance served as the beta test sites. A formal evaluation of that beta test was conducted by the National Opinion Research Center at the University of Chicago, and the results were used to refine the standards, measures, and processes that are now being used. PHAB considers its accreditation program to be driven by the practice community, with validation from the academic and research community.

The governmental entity that has the primary statutory or legal responsibility for public health—that is, state, local, tribal, and territorial health departments—is eligible for accreditation. Such entities must operate in a manner consistent with applicable federal, state, local, tribal, and territorial laws. For purposes of accreditation, the following definitions are used.

State and territorial health department The governmental body recognized in the state or territorial constitution, statutes, or regulations or established by executive order as having the primary statutory authority to promote and protect the public's health and prevent disease in humans is eligible to apply. Umbrella organizations and collaborations among state or territorial agencies can apply for accreditation if the primary entity is part of the organization or collaboration. If the state or territorial health department operates local or regional health departments, a single applicant or a number of individual applicants can apply. Compliance with local standards must be demonstrated for each local or regional unit.

Local health department The governmental body serving a jurisdiction or group of jurisdictions geographically smaller than a state that is recognized by the state's constitution, statutes, or regulations or is established by local ordinance or through formal local cooperative agreement or mutual aid and that has primary statutory authority to promote and protect the public's health and prevent disease in humans is eligible to apply. This entity may be a locally governed health department, a local entity of a centralized state health department, or a regional, county, or district health department. An entity that meets this definition can apply for accreditation jointly with other eligible local-level entities if some of the essential public health services are provided by the sharing of resources and the manner in which this occurs is clearly demonstrated.

Tribal health department The health department serving a recognized tribe that has primary statutory authority to promote and protect the public's health and prevent disease in humans is eligible to apply.[9]

The Accreditation Process

The accreditation process consists of seven basic steps, with specific activities in each. These activities are similar to other accreditation processes in other industries, with some revisions to ensure their applicability to public health.

Preapplication The health department prepares and assesses readiness checklists, views an online orientation to accreditation, and formally informs PHAB of its intent to apply. This step is for planning purposes and allows PHAB to work with health departments to ensure that they are ready to proceed with the formal process.

Application The health department submits a formal application form with three prerequisites: a community health assessment, a community health improvement plan, and a health department strategic plan. PHAB uses these prerequisites as the basis for its review. During this phase, applicants' representatives attend in-person training, which is provided to increase their overall understanding of the PHAB accreditation process.

Document selection and submission During this stage, the health department performs its own self-assessment by selecting documentation that offers the best evidence of its conformity with each measure. The selected documentation is submitted to PHAB for review by a team of peer site reviewers.

Site visit A team of peers visits the health department and prepares a report.

Accreditation decision The PHAB Board of Directors reviews the site visit report and makes a determination. If accreditation is awarded, it is valid for five years, assuming there is no significant change in the health department's operations.

Reports The accredited health department submits an annual report to PHAB, describing its progress in areas targeted for improvement or its overall quality improvement efforts.

Reaccreditation The accredited health department applies for reaccreditation in five years, and the cycle continues.[9]

Standards and Measures

The standards and measures are based on the generally accepted core functions of public health (assessment, assurance, and policy development) and the ten essential public health services. Accreditation gives reasonable assurance of the range of public health services provided by a health department. The standards refer to this broad range of work as health department processes, programs, and interventions. Although some public health departments offer mental health, substance abuse, primary care, and human and social services (including domestic violence), these activities are not considered core public health services under the framework used for accreditation purposes. Public health services may be provided directly by the health department or by another organization or entity through formal arrangements such as contracts, compacts, or memoranda of agreement. However, when public health functions are provided by another entity, by more than one entity, or through a partnership, the health department must demonstrate how the process, program, or intervention is delivered and how the health department coordinates with the other providers.[10]

PHAB's standards and measures are contained in twelve domains (see box); the first ten are similar to the ten essential public health services, and the other two were developed by PHAB to address health departments' performance related to administration and management, as well as their relationship with the governing entity. For each domain there are standards, and for each standard there are measures (e.g., measure 5.3.2 for standard 5.3 in domain 5). Each measure has been developed as either a capacity, process, or outcome measure (for those with characteristics of more than one type, the predominant characteristic is used), based on these brief definitions:

- Capacity—something that is in place.
- Process—something that must be done.
- Outcome—a change or lack of change resulting from an action or intervention. There are two subtypes: a process outcome, in which the results of a process are tracked, and a health outcome, in which the results may include health status information.[10]

The PHAB standards generally apply to every health department. The 2011 version of PHAB's standards and measures included the following for each domain.[10]

Domain 1: Conduct assessments Standards in this domain include participating in or conducting a collaborative process resulting in a comprehensive

---

PHAB's Twelve Public Health Department Accreditation Domains

1. Conduct assessments focused on population health status and health issues facing the community.
2. Investigate health problems and environmental public health hazards to protect the community.
3. Inform and educate about public health issues and functions.
4. Engage with the community to identify and solve health problems.
5. Develop public health policies and plans.
6. Enforce public health laws and regulations.
7. Promote strategies to improve access to health care services.
8. Maintain a competent public health workforce.
9. Evaluate and continuously improve processes, programs, and interventions.
10. Contribute to and apply the evidence base of public health.
11. Maintain administrative and management capacity.
12. Build a strong and effective relationship with the governing entity.

---

community health assessment; collecting and maintaining reliable, comparable, and valid data on conditions of importance to public health and on the health status of the population; analyzing the data collected to identify trends in health problems, environmental public health hazards, and the multiple determinants of health; and using the results of the analyses to develop recommendations on public health policy, processes, programs, or interventions. The significance of this domain is that the health department must demonstrate knowledge of the health status in its jurisdiction and must use that information to inform change. This domain contains the criteria by which one of the three prerequisites—the community health assessment—will be reviewed.

Domain 2: Investigate health problems and public health hazards Standards in this domain include conducting timely investigations of health problems and environmental public health hazards; containing and mitigating the problems and hazards identified; ensuring access to public health laboratory and epidemiologic expertise and the capacity to investigate and contain health problems and hazards; and maintaining an urgent and nonurgent communication plan related to these issues. These activities are significant because they enable the health department to serve in a leadership role in its community for the purpose of identifying and managing significant public health problems and hazards.

Domain 3: Inform and educate the public Standards in this domain include providing health education and health promotion activities and programs to support prevention and wellness, as well as providing information on public health issues and functions through a variety of methods to a variety of audiences. The health department must demonstrate how it both communicates with and educates its various audiences and stakeholders.

Domain 4: Engage with the community The standards in this domain include engaging with the public health system and the community to identify and address health problems through collaborative processes, along with promoting the community's understanding of and support for policies and strategies that improve public health. The significance of these standards and measures is related to the health department's demonstration of collaborative work with various sectors of the public health system toward common goals.

Domain 5: Develop public health policies and plans These standards and measures require the health department to serve as a primary and expert resource for establishing and maintaining public health practices and capacity; develop and implement an organizational strategic plan; conduct a comprehensive planning process that results in a community health improvement plan; and maintain an all-hazards emergency plan. Here, the health department works with its community members, stakeholders, and partners to develop appropriate, actionable plans aimed at improving the health status of the community it serves. These plans should be living documents that foster additional collaboration beyond their development, with measurable results. This domain contains the criteria by which two of the three prerequisites— community health improvement plan and health department strategic plan— are assessed.

Domain 6: Enforce public health laws These standards describe the health department's role in reviewing existing public health laws and working with governmental entities and elected or appointed officials to make changes as needed; educating individuals and organizations on the meaning, purpose, and benefits of public health laws; and conducting and monitoring public health enforcement activities. These standards and measures build on the increasing body of knowledge that indicates the importance of changes in law and policy for improving population health status.

Domain 7: Improve access to health care services The standards in this domain include assessing the health care capacity in the health department's jurisdiction, as well as identifying and implementing strategies to improve access to health care services. This domain defines the criteria by which a health department should work with its partners in the health care system to ensure the availability of and access to appropriate and necessary health care services. This planning should include the primary care sector, as well as the inpatient and specialty components of the health care system.

Domain 8: Maintain a competent public health workforce Health departments have an important role in ensuring that there will be a sufficient number of public health workers in the future. This domain includes standards for encouraging the development of public health workers, assessing public health staffs' competence, and addressing gaps by enabling organizational and individual staff development.

Domain 9: Evaluate and improve processes, programs, and interventions Quality improvement concepts are new to the public health field. However, the MLC initiative fostered a deeper interest in and understanding of these concepts and their application in the public health environment. This domain contains two standards: one that focuses on the use of a performance management system to improve organizational activities and interventions, and one that assesses the development and implementation of quality improvement processes in the organization. Measures for the first standard should capture how the health department reviews itself on a regular basis to determine gaps, needs, issues, and weaknesses that would lead to the second standard of implementing health department–wide quality improvement.

Domain 10: Contribute to and apply the evidence base of public health Standards in this domain describe the health department's use of the best available evidence when making informed practice decisions. They also provide a basis for reviewing how the health department promotes the use of research, best practices, and similar evidence to guide its work. The significance of this domain is that public health is a specialty built on a body of scientific knowledge that provides a firm basis for selecting the best interventions, policies, and practices that are most likely to improve the community's health status. The health department has a major role in ensuring that the scientific base for public health remains strong.

Domain 11: Maintain administrative and management capacity These standards review the basic operational infrastructure of the health department and include areas such as finance and budgeting and information systems. PHAB added this domain to the ten essential public health services as a means to review the health department's capacity to provide a solid administrative platform on which its programs can operate.

Domain 12: Engage the public health governing entity These standards describe the health department's approach to working with its governing entity as it carries out its official public health roles and responsibilities. Whether the governing entity is a board of health, the governor's office, the mayor's office, a city council, or a board of commissioners, the public health department has a role in ensuring that entity's ongoing knowledge of and engagement in public health functions that affect the population's health.

There are many methods for selecting and submitting documentation of the health department's conformity with the various measures. Some documentation may be produced by local health department staff or by the state health department for use by local health departments; others may be produced by partnerships, regional collaborations, or contracted services. The purpose of documentation is to demonstrate that the material exists and is used by the health department being reviewed. PHAB suggests the following types of documentation for each measure:

- Documentation of policies and processes: policies, procedures, protocols, standing operating procedures, manuals, flowcharts, or logic models.
- Documentation of reporting activities, data, and decisions: health data summaries, survey data summaries, data analysis, audit results, meeting agendas, committee minutes and packets, after-action evaluations, continuing education tracking reports, work plans, financial reports, or quality improvement reports.
- Documentation of distribution and other activities: e-mail, memoranda, letters, dated distribution lists, phone books, health alerts, faxes, case files, logs, attendance logs, position descriptions, performance evaluations, brochures, flyers, website screen prints, news releases, newsletters, posters, or contracts.

Documentation used to demonstrate conformity with measures should be dated within five years of the date of submission to PHAB, unless otherwise noted. Other time frames are defined as follows:

- Annually—within fourteen months of documentation submission.
- Current—within twenty-four months of documentation submission.
- Biennially—within each twenty-four-month period (at least) prior to documentation submission.
- Regular—within a preestablished schedule, as determined by the health department.
- Continuing—refers to activities that have existed for some time, are currently in existence, and will remain so in the future.[10]

Contemporary Topics Related to Public Health Accreditation

As PHAB finalized plans to open for official business in 2011, several related but tangential issues arose that may have a bearing on the success of accreditation over time. Some of these issues are discussed here.

Partnership with nonprofit hospitals to conduct community health assessments

Under new provisions of the Patient Protection and Affordable Care Act of 2010, the Internal Revenue Service (IRS) requires nonprofit hospitals to conduct community health needs assessments. Given PHAB's requirement of community health assessments and improvement plans, this creates an unprecedented opportunity for a united focus on improving public health. Proposed IRS regulations lay the groundwork for hospital systems and health departments to officially work together to conduct community health needs assessments and adopt implementation strategies to meet those needs; they also require input from the broadest segment of the population served. There is a $50,000 proposed excise tax penalty for hospital systems that do not comply.[11] Significant paradigm shifts will be necessary for a true collaborative, nonduplicative effort to occur. However, a partnership between the health care system and the public health department has the potential to benefit the community by improving its health status, and this warrants further study.

Incentives for health departments to become accredited

Since the national public health department accreditation program is voluntary, there have been many discussions about the benefits of accreditation and the return on investment. Davis and colleagues conducted a study in 2009 to determine which incentives were most likely to encourage state and local health departments to participate in a voluntary accreditation program.[12] The results indicated that financial incentives to prepare for and obtain accreditation, with a focus on improving the infrastructure and leading to quality improvement, were most likely to inspire health departments to apply for accreditation. State health departments also indicated that grant incentives would contribute to their interest in accreditation. In response, PHAB's Board of Directors developed a list of potential incentives, and it continues to work with other national partners to support the development of incentives.

Health departments are more likely to seek accreditation if the national program is credible, reliable, reasonable, and linked to current practice.

Although PHAB has made a good start in this direction, the Board of Directors has instituted regular internal checkpoints to ensure that the accreditation program continues to have these attributes at its core. Of particular interest—and not currently included in the PHAB program—is a closer connection with clinical partners in the communities served by health departments.

Statements of support for an accreditation program from various national public health partners have long been valued, but surveys now indicate that more is needed from these partners. Strong technical assistance is a key component of health department success in the accreditation program. Working with partners such as the Association of State and Territorial Health Officials, the National Association of County and City Health Officials, the National Association of Local Boards of Health, the American Public Health Association, and the National Indian Health Board, PHAB encourages specific incentive requests to all federal agencies currently and historically providing financial support to state, local, and tribal health departments. These requests should include funding for training and technical assistance for accreditation preparation, funding for accreditation application, and funding to address barriers and issues identified in the accreditation process that would lead to quality improvement in the public health agency as a whole.

Consistent with the federal government's policy on paperwork reduction and the avoidance of redundancy, the PHAB Board of Directors and its national partners recommend that the federal grant application procedure be changed to acknowledge accredited health departments and that their certificates of accreditation be accepted in lieu of required infrastructure components. Accomplishing this change would be a "win-win" for both health departments and funding agencies.

Other organizations that provide financial support to public health departments should be encouraged to acknowledge the accreditation process as one that improves the overall public health agency, and they should provide the same incentives requested of the federal government. New funding provided by both the federal government and funding foundations could be earmarked for specific work on quality improvement in those areas identified as deficient through the accreditation process.

In keeping with the push to base administrative and program decisions on knowledge and data, the PHAB Board of Directors has worked to establish an information system that provides accurate, credible data that can identify the characteristics and attributes of high-performing health departments. Having this information on a national level will allow sound management decisions in the future. High-performing health departments are expected to manage public resources more efficiently and serve their constituents more effectively.

Characteristics of high-performing health care systems that have recently been identified can inform this aspect of incentive development.

The PHAB Board of Directors has agreed to work with its national partners to better educate program managers in the federal agencies about the benefits of accreditation. It is recognized that PHAB's accreditation standards and measures are not program specific. However, it is also recognized that public health programs require a strong "core" public health foundation on which to operate. Aligning programmatic expectations with PHAB's assurances related to accreditation outcomes has the potential to reduce duplication in program review efforts and to ensure a solid base for public health programs. In the future, accredited health departments applying for grants from the federal government or from private foundations and other grant-making organizations could be rewarded with additional funds (based on their accreditation), especially when competition for funds exists.

Although all health departments need some assistance in preparing for accreditation, both extremely small and extremely large health departments require a different type of assistance than midsize health departments. The PHAB Board of Directors has worked with its national partner organizations and funders to ascertain the specific needs of small health departments to provide incentives for them to be accredited. The needs and issues associated with large, complex health departments are currently being addressed through one of PHAB's think-tank efforts, and recommendations for incentives will be forthcoming.[13]

The challenges of measuring organizational performance

Because the standards and measures of the accreditation program are based on former work, such as the NPHPSP, they are assumed to be valid measures of health department performance. In 2003 Beaulieu and associates conducted a content and criterion validity study of the NPHPSP and determined its validity for measuring local and state public health system performance, within the context of the psychometrics utilized.[14] However, appropriate psychometric assessments for the PHAB standards and measures need to be conducted as relevant data from accredited health departments become available, and adjustments in the measurement criteria will be made accordingly.

Contributing to the evidence base for public health

An interesting challenge in developing an accreditation program has been the lack of evidence that accreditation will make a difference in identified outcomes. In a working paper prepared for the Robert Wood Johnson Foundation, Mays reflected on whether accreditation can work in public health, based on observations of the impact of accreditation in other industries.[15] To ensure that accreditation data contribute to the evidence base for public health, PHAB developed an accreditation research agenda that has been distributed to public health systems researchers and potential funders.[16] The research agenda is quite lengthy and detailed, but a few of its major questions include:

- What are the characteristics of accredited health departments?
- Do the PHAB standards and measures capture the most meaningful information to measure the performance of health departments?
- What is the relationship between accreditation status and the management of public health programs such as tobacco prevention, obesity reduction and prevention, and environmental public health (to name a few)?
- Does accreditation contribute to better health outcomes?

One of the most important features of an accreditation program is a credible information system containing data that can be used to answer these and many other research questions and thus contribute to the evidence base for public health.

Relationship to quality improvement

Although quality improvement has been embraced by the health care system, the concept is new to the public health field. A definition of quality improvement in public health was developed by the Accreditation Coalition and published in 2010. Specifically, it describes how the concept can be used in a public health setting: "Quality improvement in public health is the use of a deliberate and defined improvement process, such as Plan-Do-Check-Act, which is focused on activities that are responsive to community needs and improving population health. It refers to a continuous and ongoing effort to achieve measurable improvements in the efficiency, effectiveness, performance, accountability, outcomes, and other indicators of quality in services or processes which achieve equity and improve the health of the community."[17] In addition, the Department of Health and Human Services has issued a document that delineates the priority areas for quality improvement in public health. This model describes quality improvement aims, as well as primary and secondary drivers of quality in the public health setting.[18]

During the beta test conducted by PHAB, the thirty sites planned and implemented quality improvement initiatives based on needs identified during the mock accreditation process. Health departments reported reduced times for conducting environmental health inspections, better customer satisfaction, lower clinic no-show rates, and increased community engagement in the work of the public health department. Clearly, public health still has significant developmental work to do to create a sustained culture of quality improvement.

PHAB's assumption is that high-performing health departments employing the latest innovations in public health science and best practices will positively affect the health of the communities they serve. Development of a credible system of information that describes the processes, interventions, and infrastructure required to decrease infant mortality, improve epidemiologic surveillance, strengthen health education for multicultural neighborhoods, and foster better communication of health laws and regulations will certainly help transform public health and put it in a better position to positively impact the health status of its citizens.

Notes

1. Shattuck L. *Report of the Sanitary Commission of Massachusetts.* Boston: Dutton and Wentworth; 1850. http://www.deltaomega.org/shattuck.pdf. Accessed June 15, 2011.

2. Cooperation in public health administration in the small community. *JAMA.* 1914;63(14):1207–1208. http://jama.ama-assn.org/content/LXIII/14/1207.extract. Accessed June 15, 2011.

3. Halverson W. A twenty-five year review of the work of the Committee on Administrative Practice. *Am J Public Health.* 1945;35(12):1253–1259.

4. Turnock BJ, Barnes P. History will be kind [commentary]. *J Public Health Manage Pract.* 2007;13(4):337–341.

5. Institute of Medicine. *The Future of Public Health.* Washington, DC: National Academies Press; 1988.

6. Institute of Medicine. *The Future of the Public's Health in the 21st Century.* Washington, DC: National Academies Press; 2003.

7. *Final Recommendations for a Voluntary National Accreditation Program for State and Local Public Health Departments.* Exploring Accreditation Project Report. Washington, DC; 2006.

8. Beitsch LM, Thielen L, Mays G, et al. *The Multistate Learning Collaborative. States as Laboratories: Informing the National Public Health Accreditation Dialogue.* Robert Wood Johnson Foundation; 2006. http://www.rwjf.org/pr/product .jsp?id=15409. Accessed June 8, 2009.

9. Public Health Accreditation Board. *Version 1.0 Guide to National Public Health Department Accreditation.* Application period 2011–2012. Alexandria, VA; 2011.

10. Public Health Accreditation Board. *Version 1.0 Standards and Measures.* Application period 2011–2012. Alexandria, VA; 2011.

11. Internal Revenue Service. Proposed rules and regulations. http://www.irs.gov/pub/irs-drop/n-10-39.pdf. Accessed July 8, 2011.

12. Davis M, Cannon M, Corso L, Lenaway D, Baker E. Incentives to encourage participation in the national public health accreditation model: A systematic review. *Am J Public Health.* 2009;99(9):1–7.

13. Public Health Accreditation Board. Incentives for public health accreditation. Unpublished policy paper. February 2010. http://www.phaboard.org. Accessed May 21, 2011.

14. Beaulieu F, Scutchfield FD, Kelly AV. Content and criterion validity evaluation of National Public Health Performance Standards measurement instruments. *Public Health Rep.* 2003;118(6):508–517.

15. Mays G. Can accreditation work in public health? Lessons learned from other service industries. Working paper. Robert Wood Johnson Foundation; November 30, 2004. http://www.phaboard.org/assets/documents/Accreditationinpublichealth_GlenMays.pdf. Accessed June 15, 2011.

16. Public Health Accreditation Board. Public health accreditation research agenda. Unpublished policy paper. May 2011. http://www.phaboard.org. Accessed June 25, 2011.

17. Riley WJ, Moran JW, Corso LC, Beitsch LM, Bialek R, Cofsky A. Defining quality improvement in public health. *J Public Health Manage Pract.* 2010;16(1):5–7.

18. Honore P, Wright D, Berwick D, Clancy CM, Lee P, Nowinski J, Koh H. Creating a framework for getting quality into the public health system. *Health Aff.* 2011;30(4):737–745.

8

Contemporary Issues in Scientific Communication and Public Health Education

Charlotte S. Seidman, William M. Silberg, and Kevin Patrick

This chapter addresses both the long tradition of and the rapidly changing environment for communicating information that is essential to public health and preventive medicine research, policy, and practice. As editors of the *American Journal of Preventive Medicine*, we deal with this on a daily basis. But we rarely have the opportunity to step back and reflect on the process of our work, its historical basis, where it is now, and where it is likely to be in the coming years. Unlike many domains of science that thrive on highly specialized research papers that present findings of no immediate import to practice or policy, some of the best research in public health is intended to have an immediate impact on problems of major importance to entire populations of individuals. How do we detect outbreaks of serious infectious disease sooner than we have before? Once detected, how are such outbreaks interrupted and curtailed to minimize death and disability? How do we characterize the problem of adverse childhood experiences and their sequelae and intervene to prevent them? What policy interventions work best to reduce tobacco-related disease? What are the costs of childhood obesity, and who bears them? All these questions represent situations in which scientific and technical knowledge must be linked via communication strategies as quickly as possible with policy and program formulation. Moreover, much of this information needs to be accessible to the general public because solutions are rarely if ever successfully implemented without its acceptance. This dual allegiance, professional and public, defines much of the way we think about our work, and as we emphasize in this chapter, new media technologies provide both opportunities and challenges for communication in this arena.

After reviewing the roots of scientific communication, this chapter examines the changing landscape of scientific communication and its implications for researchers, policy makers, and practitioners. We also focus on issues that are relevant to the public side of our work by addressing health literacy and health numeracy, theories and methods of health communication, and recent trends in the democratization (for lack of a better word) of scientific communication via the increasingly pervasive web of electronic, mobile, and social media within which we all spend a great part of our lives.

Background

Communication and publication are inextricably linked. The publishing of information is one way humans communicate. Throughout history, advances in publication methods have determined the ease (or not) with which communication occurs. Scientific communication is currently undergoing a transformation from traditional media to new media, and from a professionally mediated ex cathedra model to one in which the communication of research findings and their implications is increasingly concurrent—to both public health professionals and the general public simultaneously. Although this process can rapidly provide information of immediate relevance to users, it can also dilute the validation process provided by professional mediation. Moreover, low barriers to entry for e-communicators can lead to a much higher background "noise" level, which can be distracting to professional communication and even undercut valid information that is important to the public's health.

A Brief History of Communication

"The history of communication is mankind's search for ways to improve upon shouting."[1] In antiquity, many human activities were based on the need to communicate—for example, running from town to town to disseminate news and the use of town criers—and many early inventions came about for the same reason: to spread the word to others across space. The need for portable writing tools thus became critical. Carving on stone worked for local communication, but portable tools were needed for longer-distance communication. Smoke signals worked fairly well, but their distance was limited; in addition, they were nonverbal and could not communicate the nuances of messages.

The advent of writing tools and papyrus was one of the first major leaps into mass communication. Messages could now be shared, kept, and even

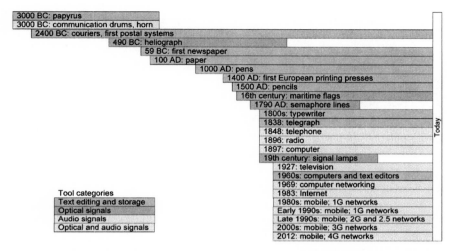

Figure 8.1. Time line of communication tools. *Sources:* By Mhd Alaa Al Khourdaje. Based on Michael A, Salter B. *Mobile Marketing: Achieving Competitive Advantage through Wireless Technology.* Amsterdam: Elsevier; 2006.

stored, but still within a limited physical setting. The first recorded courier and postal system was noted in 2400 BC; the first newspaper in 59 BC. Paper as we know it today was invented around AD 100, while pencils took another 1,400 years to appear on the scene (figure 8.1).[2] Of all the innovative communication tools developed before the Christian era, only the postal system and newspapers survived into the modern era. Most of the communication tools created in the Christian era are still used today, although they have been altered to "stay in the market" as they converged with later tools.

To successfully move messages from one place to another, passageways had to be built. Expanding roads to facilitate messages' moving from one place to another became the goal. Better roads, fresher horses, and stopping places along the way all became critical to the process.

At the same time, the process of printing evolved—from papyrus to paper, from scribes to movable print. And the process of communication evolved in tandem—semaphore flags, the typewriter, telegraph, telephone, radio, computer, television, and computer networking.

Humanity's need to communicate is an outcome (indeed, a requirement) of its social nature. "No man is an island" may be an overused adage, but that should not distract from its basic truth. Humans need to communicate to live and to thrive. As humanity progressed through the centuries, so did the need for more sophisticated means of communication. When the population of the world was limited to central Asia and Africa and then spread into Europe, communication needs were more easily met; as the population expanded to all the continents, meeting these needs became more of a challenge.

Societal typology also played a role in communication. In the early years, the "lower class" was not expected to read, but this changed as each society progressed through the stages of geopolitical development. Whereas reading and communication were once the "rights of the rich," the advent of movable print and book binding and the mass marketing of literature (as well as social reform) changed the face of literacy and thus communication skills.

Although the tools for communicating have changed over the centuries, the basic need is the same (see box).[3] Humanity communicates to stay connected, to be in the know, to learn, to grow. Humans communicate because it is a basic need for existence. Communication skills have matured as humanity has matured. From smoke signals and beating on drums to wireless technologies, the evolution of communication has demonstrated the creative genius of humans at their best (figure 8.2).

The Importance of Communication

Information dissemination: It is owing to the process of communication that we are able to send and receive information. Various mass media are an important communication tool for information dissemination.

Expressing emotions and ideas: Imagine a life without expressing yourself through words (spoken and written), expressions, and even arts and crafts or painting, music, or dance. Communication helps people express their ideas and emotions.

Education: Communication plays an important role in the process of imparting knowledge. Communication is instrumental in the process of education because it helps educators and students interact.

Building relationships: Communication facilitates dialogue, the exchange of ideas, and the expression of human emotions between people. Thus, it helps build and maintain relationships—whether it is business communication or interpersonal communication.

Entertainment: Movies, music, television shows, theater, and even anecdotes narrated by people are types of communication that entertain us.

Decision making: Communication helps in the process of decision making, whether individual or group decision making.

Source: Michael A, Salter B. *Mobile Marketing: Achieving Competitive Advantage through Wireless Technology.* Amsterdam: Elsevier, 2006.

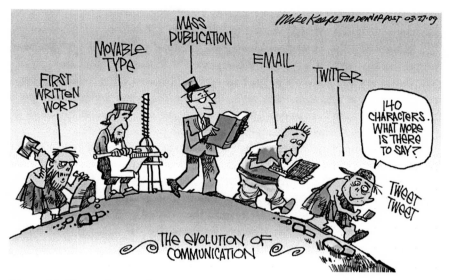

Figure 8.2. The evolution of communication. *Source:* Mike Keefe, *Denver Post* and In-Toon.com. Reprinted by permission.

A Brief History of Scientific Publication

In 1517, when Martin Luther presented his famous ninety-five theses to the archbishop (and probably not by nailing them to the door), the action of printing and distributing the work made the controversy one of the first in history to be aided by the printing press.[4] The distribution of information has been around since the beginning of humanity, but it was the 1440 invention of the printing press that had the most marked impact on publishing per se until the present time. Movable print and the later invention of the rotary press (in 1843) allowed for mass printing, which led to the speedier dissemination of information.

It was not until the seventeenth century that the first scientific papers were published. These papers were not yet combined into journals; rather, they were just an individual's thoughts and comments. The first formal journals, one British and one French, appeared around the 1670s and consisted of the transactions of scholarly societies. Prior to that time, lectures and books were the main means of scientific communication (although some surgical "books" date to ancient Egypt). Two of the oldest formal journals are the *New England Journal of Medicine* (*NEJM*) and the *Lancet,* which started printing in 1812 and 1823, respectively. The *NEJM* started as a quarterly for both medicine and surgery and adopted its current name in 1928. The *Journal of the American Medical Association* (*JAMA*) started publishing in 1883.

At the time the *Lancet* was launched, medical practice in England was fundamentally corrupt.[5] Thomas Wakely wanted to use his publication to expose that corruption and chose the name *Lancet* because it is a medical instrument used to cut and drain abscesses. Over the years, the *Lancet* has been a leader in launching campaigns against corruption and exposing mistakes. It has influenced not only medical practice but also policy and politics.

The combined inventions of the computer and the Internet have had the most influence on modern publishing. The concept of *publishing* itself has been forced to change, to adapt to the online-only publication of scientific articles, and to accept as "published" works that are shared in the networked world. Publishing has moved well beyond the printed page and will continue to evolve as a new generation of scientific researchers assumes responsibility for maintaining the literature base.

So the passageways of old—the expanding roadways that facilitated the movement of messages from one place to another—have been replaced by the passageways for today's technology—the Internet and the World Wide Web, with their blogs and social networks, and wireless communication technologies.

Reader Expectations

Regardless of the format in which scientific information is presented, the end users—that is, the readers—are the ultimate judge of the usefulness of the material. Readers will continue to be the audience of record of any published work, and they will have to be appeased by the processes and formats of scientific literature. Reader expectations will continue to drive the way material is presented in the scientific literature. Readers expect material to be presented in a certain order, and they may be confused and unable to follow the material if there is any variation in that format. For better or worse, the tradition of writing a scientific paper and the structure it takes have become de rigueur for both authors and readers.[6]

Readers expect correct grammar, proper syntax, and punctuation. Peer review of the content of published material is just as important for the online delivery of scientific material as for formal printed versions, as it maintains the clear and unambiguous presentation of research findings.

Digital Tools in Professional Publishing

Electronic publishing (or e-publishing) is a new type of information dissemination. It refers to the online and Web-based publication of works of fiction and scientific articles, as well as the development of digital libraries and catalogs. In the context of scientific communication, e-publishing is the presentation of material only in an electronic (nonpaper) form—from its first write-up to its publication or dissemination; such material is not previously printed text that has been adapted or retooled for electronic delivery.

Over the past fifteen years or so, many established print journals have developed electronic approaches to disseminate their peer-reviewed and edited "published" articles. By 2006, almost all scientific journals had established electronic versions, and a number of them have moved entirely to electronic publication. Other journals, whether spin-offs of established print journals or specifically created as electronic publications, exist to promote the rapid dissemination and availability of information on the Internet. As a result of this transformation, many academic libraries now buy the electronic versions of most journals and purchase paper copies of only the most important or most popular titles.

An important construct of electronic publication is the recognition that such material has been officially published. This has been managed through the creation of the digital object identifier (DOI), which identifies and recognizes intellectual content and enables the automated management of media. Once a scientific paper has been assigned a DOI, it is considered published and can be located online using only that identifier. The system is managed by the International DOI Foundation, an open-membership consortium including both commercial and noncommercial partners.[7]

With print-based publishing, there are generally delays of several months between the time an article is written and its publication in a journal. With electronic publishing, many journals now publish final papers as soon as they are ready, without waiting for the assembly of a complete issue. In many fields in which even greater speed is desired, such as physics, the role of the journal has largely been replaced by preprint databases such as http://arXiv.org. Almost all such articles are eventually published in traditional journals, however, which still play an important part in maintaining quality control, archiving, and establishing scientific credit.

In tandem with the move to electronic publication is the migration to online processes for peer review, copyediting, page makeup, and other steps in the process. Electronic publishing of scientific journals has been accomplished without compromising the standards of the refereed, peer-review process. And electronically published scientific journals often cost less and are more accessible, especially to scientists and practitioners working in undeveloped and underdeveloped countries.

Advances in information technology and networking now support two additional phenomena that merit close attention in the public health and pre-vention community: data sharing and open access before peer review. Al-though the vast majority of journals in the health-related disciplines continue to follow the standard processes of peer review followed by publication, some advocate a rapid release of source data to researchers and, if appropriate, to the public without peer review.

Data sharing can serve two purposes. First, it can increase the transpar-ency of the research experiment itself, rendering all aspects of a study—its design, measures, initial hypotheses, plans for analysis, and methods of data collection—understandable to users. It is then up to the users to make con-clusions about the validity and relevance of the data to them. Second, data sharing supports the use of data beyond what was initially envisioned in the primary study. Any given set of researchers might ask different questions of a given data set. And researchers in the future might come up with totally new questions to ask of the same data set. There is even an expression for this: To-day's noise may be tomorrow's signal!

In response, some journals have chosen to play a role in data sharing. For example, the *British Medical Journal* (*BMJ*) now asks authors to include a data-sharing statement to explain which additional data from their stud-ies, if any, are available, to whom, and how. They may be willing to share only supplementary material or the complete data set; the data may be available only on request, accessible online with a password, or openly accessible to all with a link on http://www.bmj.com—perhaps after a clearly stated period of personal use.[8] Data sharing is also increasingly recommended by funders such as the National Institutes of Health (NIH), which may have an inter-est in maximizing the value of their investments in research. Grant propos-als to NIH often require a data-sharing plan and an up-front agreement that data will be placed in a common repository for use by others after a certain period.

Open access before peer review, although related to data sharing, can serve a different purpose. In this case, the findings of a study, including the interpretation and analysis of source data, are released before being submit-ted to the standard editorial and peer-review process. The intent is to bypass any form of judgment that might constrain the dissemination of findings. Tra-ditionally, a community of scientists arrives at the "truth" by independently verifying new observations. In this time-honored process, journals serve two functions: evaluative and editorial. In their evaluative function, they winnow out research that does not stand up to independent verification through the process of peer review. This is usually done in either a single- or double-blind fashion, whereby the reviewers do not know who the authors are and/or the authors do not know who the reviewers are. The rationale for this anonymity is to increase candor in the process and reduce the likelihood of animosity between the parties. In their editorial function, journals try to ensure transparent (that is, clear, complete, and unambiguous) and objective descriptions of the research. Both the evaluative and editorial functions go largely unnoticed by the public—the former draws public attention only when a journal publishes fraudulent research.[9] Although many believe that these functions play a critical role in the progress of science, some find that they stifle the growth of knowledge by tending to support the status quo and undervaluing true breakthroughs in science because the reviewers and editors are incapable of "getting" everything a paper might convey.

For the foreseeable future, electronic publishing will exist alongside paper publishing. Output to a screen is important for browsing and searching, but it is not yet well adapted for extensive reading. While efforts continue to find a medium that supports electronic writing and reading characteristics that can replace paper, print copies of certain information continue to have high levels of use. Formats suitable for both reading on paper and manipulating by computer will need to share common elements if they are to convey equivalent information to users. The reality of new media is that the field is moving quickly and in many directions, and the interested reader would be well advised to follow these developments with an open—and critical—mind.

Health Communication

Health communication can be defined in many ways. According to *Healthy People 2010*, it is "the art and technique of informing, influencing, and motivating individual, institutional, and public audiences about important health issues. The scope of health communication includes disease prevention, health promotion, healthcare policy, and the business of health care as well as enhancement of the quality of life and health of individuals within the community."[10] Cline defines it as "an area of theory, research and practice related to understanding and influencing the interdependence of communication (symbolic interaction in the forms of messages and meanings) and health-related beliefs, behaviors and outcomes."[11] Schiavo calls health communication "a multifaceted and multidisciplinary approach to reach different audiences and share health-related information with the goal of influencing, engaging and supporting individuals, communities, health professionals, special groups, policymakers and the public to champion, introduce, adopt, or sustain a behavior, practice or policy that will ultimately improve health outcomes."[12]

Background

Health communication is the process of using focused communications and educational strategies to inform and influence individual and community decisions that can affect personal and public health. A well-established field that has generated a substantial body of supporting professional literature, health communication is widely recognized as integral to campaigns to promote health and wellness generally, as well as to reduce morbidity and mortality associated with particularly burdensome acute and chronic diseases.[13-17] It is also an increasingly important element in the health policy sphere, given the highly complex process of translating policy into practice and practice into measurable and positive public health outcomes.

Health communication has been affected by the same fast-moving developments in information technology and media that have transformed many aspects of our lives. There is an evolving realization that health communication and education increasingly occur within and across multiple delivery vehicles and venues that are both professional and consumer oriented, particularly the growing number of Internet-based and digital channels that interconnect public and professionals, often on a nearly real-time basis.

This dramatic change in the traditional health communication paradigm presents public health professionals with enormous opportunities to craft and deliver more customized health promotion and disease prevention campaigns more cost-effectively, particularly to communities that may be difficult to reach because of cultural, economic, or other sociodemographic factors. But it also poses tremendous challenges for health professionals, given the sometimes daunting levels of background noise that can compete with efforts to deliver accurate, targeted messages designed to change personal health behaviors and improve a population's health. Indeed, as Neuhauser and others have noted, although there is "substantial epidemiological evidence that widespread adoption of specific behavior changes can significantly improve population health . . . health communication efforts, while well intentioned, have often failed to engage people to change behavior within the complex contexts of their lives."[18]

Communication theory, research, and interventions

Communication theory draws from a broad range of social and behavioral science disciplines and is the interface between health communication research and health communication interventions. Communication research is used to develop and test theories of communication, information processing, and human behavior. These theories seek to explain how and why audiences process health information, the impact of communication and information on behavior, and how factors in the social and physical environment mediate the relationship between communication and behavior. Theories that have useful predictive and prescriptive power (such as social cognitive theory, the theory of reasoned action, stages of change theory, theories of risk perception, and framing theory) are powerful assets in planning successful public health communication interventions.[12, 15, 17]

This theoretical and research foundation underlies the concept of health communication, defined by the National Cancer Institute (NCI) and the Centers for Disease Control and Prevention (CDC) as "the study and use of communication strategies to inform and influence individual and community decisions that enhance health."[13] Effective applications of these strategies adhere closely to basic principles of strategic communication. This is the systematic process of identifying key messages and audiences and establishing an integrated framework of tools and channels to connect and engage the two on an ongoing basis for the purpose of achieving a specific goal (or goals), monitoring progress toward that goal, and changing approaches as results dictate. One cannot overstate the importance of such a systematic approach that includes the explicit identification of goals and target audiences; clear, consistent, and appropriate messaging; and metrics for gauging success. The NCI and CDC underscore the importance of this integrated, multipronged approach, noting that "successful health communication programs involve more than the production of messages and materials. They use research-based strategies to shape the products and determine the channels that deliver them to the right intended audiences."[10, 18]

As the NCI and others have noted, effective health communication initiatives utilize and leverage a combination of tactics and approaches, including public education (sharing tailored health information with the public), social marketing (designing health messages and programs to change the health behaviors of the target audience, and involving that audience in the planning process), and media advocacy (using media strategically to reframe issues, shape public discussion, or build support for a policy, point of view, or environmental change). Media can be particularly powerful in this regard; as Hornik notes, media coverage and media accuracy "may play no less a role in the process of behavior change than do formal efforts at influencing behavior through educational efforts."[19]

Many researchers have commented on the unique and crucial role that communication plays in health promotion and public health and education programs. In his essay for the online *Encyclopedia of Public Health*, for example, Maibach provides a cogent and important look at health communication and the theories that support the translation of health research into interventions to improve public health (see box).[20]

Research questions that have attracted considerable interest include whether bias in news coverage leads the public to worry excessively about rare health risks, while ignoring more prevalent health risks; whether people process health information in systematically biased ways that contribute to "irrational" decision making; and whether the news media tend to "frame" public health issues in a manner that obscures the true nature of the problem, thereby obscuring the most promising solutions.[16, 21-24] Answers to these and other research questions are used to develop communication interventions to improve health outcomes. For example, the NIH (in partnership with health professionals' associations, voluntary health agencies, and pharmaceutical companies) conducted a communication campaign that contributed to a more than 60 percent reduction in deaths from stroke, while campaigns conducted around the world during the 1990s led to rapid and dramatic reductions (50 to 80 percent) in mortality from sudden infant death syndrome (SIDS).

Public health professionals face numerous challenges in crafting such campaigns. Accurate information about health is often lost amid the background noise generated by those with commercial, advocacy, political, or other interests who are intent on delivering their own messages on health topics. An increasingly wired public and the often bizarre dynamics of an insatiable news industry can feed this level of clutter. Of additional concern is the challenge of health literacy, which is known to vary, based on a range of sociodemographic and educational factors.

Health literacy

Health literacy is the capacity to obtain, process, and understand the basic health information and services needed to make appropriate health decisions.[6] Nearly 90 percent of U.S. adults have difficulty using the everyday health information routinely distributed in health care facilities or through the media. Limited health literacy is associated with poorer health outcomes and higher health care costs. Limited health literacy affects people's ability to use health information, adopt healthy behaviors, and act on important public health alerts.[6] If standard health messages are written at a level that is beyond the comprehension of the people for whom they are intended, that information will be useless. The writer must take into consideration the audience and adapt the message accordingly.

Failure to adapt the message to fit the audience is a particular barrier to effective health communication in some of the very communities that could benefit most from health promotion and disease prevention initiatives.

Principles for Effective Public Health Communication

Public health communication is inherently pragmatic. It embraces theories, organizing frameworks, and implementation tactics from many different professional and academic disciplines. Four of the more important aspects of public health communication are media campaigns, social marketing, risk communication, and media advocacy. Although these differ considerably, particularly with regard to their organizing frameworks, they share some underlying principles of effective communication:

Know your audience. The first and most important step in communication planning is to gain as much insight as possible into the target audience. This is done primarily by conducting original audience research (e.g., focus groups, surveys), assessing the results of previous communication efforts, and drawing from theories of communication and behavior change.

Focus on the right objective. The strategies and tactics of a communication intervention will differ, depending on the stated objective (e.g., informed decision making, persuasion, policy change advocacy). A clear statement of objectives focuses and enhances all other elements of the communication planning process.

Determine which information is of greatest value. For a variety of reasons, public health communication campaigns are always limited in the amount of information they can successfully convey. Therefore, a critical step is to determine which information will have the greatest value in achieving the stated objective. The ideal (albeit rare) scenario is one in which a single powerful idea is sufficient to motivate and enable members of the target audience to embrace the campaign's objective.

Convey simple, clear messages many times, through many sources. After the information with the greatest value has been identified, communication planners must determine how to convey that information simply, clearly, often, and by many trusted sources. Message repetition is an important element of program success. Audiences tend to process information incrementally over time. When the message is stated simply and clearly, when it is repeated often enough, and when it is stated by many trusted sources, audience members are more likely to learn and embrace the message.

Sources: Maibach EW. Communication for health. *Encyclopedia of Public Health.* http://www.enotes.com/public-health-encyclopedia; Committee on Communication for Behavior Change in the 21st Century, Institute of Medicine of the National Academies. *Speaking of Health: Assessing Health Communications Strategies for Diverse Populations.* Washington, DC: National Academies Press; 2002.

Nutbeam is among those who frame health literacy as a public health goal that is crucial to empowerment and notes that improving health literacy requires "more personal forms of communication, and community-based educational outreach, as well as the political content of health education, focused on better equipping people to overcome structural barriers to health."[25, 26]

Although its roots date back centuries (to Cotton Mather's smallpox vaccination campaign in colonial America) if not millennia (to Aristotle's theories of persuasion), the field of public health communication is very much an outgrowth of contemporary social conditions.[20] Demographic, social, and technological trends over the second half of the twentieth century made the value of high-quality health information, and thus the value of effectively delivering that information for the purpose of improving health, increasingly clear.

Both today and in the future, public health communication is likely to be integrated in core public health disciplines, especially health education and promotion. Other disciplines, including epidemiology, health policy, occupational health, environmental health, international health, and health services research, are likely to increasingly appreciate and value both the fundamental importance of communications processes and the potential of effective communication to improve the health of the public.

New tools and new channels in a high-tech era

Although many of the basic principles of effective health communication have not changed substantially over the years, channels of information delivery and audience engagement have changed in dramatic and transformative ways. Over the past fifteen years, there have been unprecedented shifts in how both professional and public audiences seek, access, and utilize health information. These innovations have pervaded the way research is conducted, medicine is practiced, policy is made, and the public engages with health care professionals and one another.

Traditional media—print and broadcast—have long been critical mechanisms for disseminating health information to the general public, and they have been a focal point of many traditional public health communication and health education initiatives. These approaches remain important components of such efforts, but the Internet has provided health professionals with a powerful new vehicle for reaching large public audiences with tailored health messages in a highly cost-effective fashion. The more recent development of digital communications channels, especially social media platforms such as Facebook and Twitter and the growing network of health-oriented blogs, has provided even more opportunities.[27-29]

Although health information and health-related communities have existed in various online environments for several decades, the development of the World Wide Web in the mid-1990s provided the spark that led to today's ubiquitous digital health communication. Virtually all professional health and medical publishers, institutions, agencies, and organizations have robust online components. Digital technologies have also allowed the development of information providers that were once considered upstarts but have now become mainstream and highly influential (e.g., Medscape, Up To Date). Concurrently, a wide range of online consumer health resources has sprung up, including commercial (e.g., WebMD); nonprofit institution–based (e.g., Mayo Clinic); government-based (e.g., Medline Plus, Healthfinder); and patient-generated (e.g., Association of Cancer Online Resources, Patients Like Me) sources.

Adoption of these new communication technologies has been rapid and broad. The Pew Internet and American Life Project, for example, reported in May 2011 that almost 60 percent of American adults used the Internet in 2010 to seek information about health topics, such as a specific disease or treatment. It further noted that 11 percent of adults use social networks to interact with friends on health care issues, and 7 percent seek health information through these same channels.

These new technologies are being used not only to enhance standard professional-to-professional exchanges but also to fuel what might be considered more "disruptive" consumer-to-consumer and consumer-to-professional interactions. By allowing people to reach across the boundaries that traditionally separated health professionals and the general public, these technologies have the opportunity to gauge, in close to real time, how well public health messages are being received, processed, and "heard." This unprecedented level of audience engagement and monitoring also offers the chance to revise, reshape, retailor, or resend health messages to make them more effective. It is this aspect of digital health communication that, as Neuhauser and Kreps put it, "may have great potential to promote desired behavior changes through unique features such as mass customization, interactivity and convenience. . . . However, we have much to learn about whether the technical promise of e-health communication will be effective within the social reality of how diverse people communicate and change in the modern world."[29]

Social media and increased connectivity

The health communication landscape has been dramatically changed by the emergence of social media channels designed not just to disseminate information in a traditional one-way fashion but also to encourage engagement and interaction among and between communities of interest. These channels include the well-known social networks Facebook and Twitter; the large number of blogs used by professionals and consumers to offer their own perspectives on topics of interest and encourage comments; and technical tools designed to enhance collaborative content development, research, and problem solving, such as wikis and various "open innovation" platforms.

There are seemingly endless opportunities to leverage these emerging technologies and media, as well as to better leverage traditional media, to help individuals and families adopt healthier lifestyles, gain information on health promotion and disease management, and interact more effectively with health care professionals. Indeed, many professionals have begun to experiment with these new channels as integral components of health communication and education initiatives. These efforts are sometimes referred to as the Health 2.0 or Medicine 2.0 movement—a nod to the term Web 2.0, coined by technology media pioneer Tim O'Reilly in 2004 to characterize a new generation of Web development and utilization marked by an emphasis on information sharing, collaboration, community building, open data standards, and user-generated and -mediated content and applications.

Among the more notable Web 2.0 constructs is "crowdsourcing," the notion that expertise on any given topic is not limited to a small group of recognized "authorities" who share wisdom in a top-down fashion; rather, such expertise is widely distributed within—and thus available from—numerous communities of interest, some of which are nontraditional or unexpected. This many-to-many or many-to-some approach, driven by the concept that multiple contributions produce a corpus of work that is far more useful than that which any single or small group of experts could produce alone, undergirds such Web 2.0 developments as Wikipedia and the open innovation, problem-solving challenge movement.

In the last few years, publishers, academic medical centers and other health care institutions, government agencies, philanthropic organizations, and advocacy groups have adopted many of these tools and approaches. Some sectors have embraced them more rapidly and more fully than others, given their still-evolving business models and a lingering reticence in some disciplines to accept the transparency they demand, but the trend is clear. A few prominent examples are listed here:

- The Department of Health and Human Services (DHHS) has created the Center for New Media (http://newmedia.hhs.gov) and "open government" initiatives (http://www.hhs.gov/open) that offer access to a range of health databases so that interested developers can design applications to make them more useful to researchers, clinicians, policy makers, and the public. DHHS, along with the NIH and many of its constituents, promotes this effort through a number of developer "challenges," with cash prizes awarded to the winning submissions. Numerous DHHS agencies utilize social media channels as part of specific health education and communication campaigns; among the more prominent is the AIDS website (http://www.aids.gov).

- The CDC, long a good source of health communication and social marketing tools through its CDC Gateway to Health Communication and Social Marketing Practice (http://www.cdc.gov/healthcommunication), has created a CDC Social Media Toolkit (http://www.cdc.gov/healthcommunication/ToolsTemplates/SocialMediaToolkit_BM.pdf).
- The Mayo Clinic launched the Center for Social Media (socialmedia.mayoclinic.org) in 2010. It is probably the most proactive of the major medical centers, aggressively promoting social media not only as an important element of its health information, education, and communication activities but also as an avenue for enhanced clinical practice and medical education.
- The giant professional publisher Elsevier opened up its catalog of scientific content and challenged developers to create applications to improve researcher productivity and work flow. Winners of the challenge will be able to market their applications through Elsevier's global database platform.

If professional adoption of these tools has been dramatic, adoption by consumers—especially those with particular interests in health care issues, such as members of various chronic disease communities and advocacy organizations—has been breathtaking. Indeed, adoption by the professional community is likely being driven in no small part by pressure from the new generation of "e-patients." In this case, "e" can also mean empowered, because today's health care consumers are using an array of digital tools to proactively manage their own health; they are connecting with others with similar concerns to share information, promote an aggressive research agenda, and push for wider adoption of clinical best practices. Facebook, Twitter, and other social networking platforms have been particularly useful in supporting these initiatives.

The concurrent explosive growth in wireless technology has provided an extra level of connectivity, interactivity, and audience access to numerous health communication and other initiatives. With the nearly universal availability of cell phone service in the developed world and its widespread availability in the developing world as well, market opportunities for such applications are likely to expand rapidly. The trend is already apparent:

- Forty percent of Americans own smart phones (Nielsen Company, September 2011).
- More than 80 percent of physicians will use smart phones in 2012 (Manhattan Research, May 2011).
- The mobile health applications market will hit $1.7 billion by 2014 (Chilmark Research, November 2010).
- Users downloaded 600 million health applications in 2010 (Pyramid Research, December 2010).

It is no longer necessary to be tethered to a desktop computer to deliver information and obtain user feedback. Many health communication initiatives can now be delivered to targeted audiences in real time at the point of use. But the growing power of mobile devices—smart phones, tablet computers, and the like—to facilitate two-way data transfer, augmented by audio, video, and geopositioning technology, has created a robust and unprecedented platform for health communication and public health applications, from the simple to the highly sophisticated. Examples range from text-based health promotion and patient education services to smart phone–based health status monitoring, infectious disease surveillance, and emergency preparedness applications.

As promising as these new technologies are, they also pose substantial challenges: they tend to level the playing field between professionals and the public and operate in a culture of openness and interaction that not all health care professionals find familiar or comfortable. *Healthy People 2020* notes: "Social media and emerging technologies promise to blur the line between expert and peer health information. Monitoring and assessing the impact of these new media, including mobile health, on public health will be challenging. Equally challenging will be helping health professionals and the public adapt to the changes in healthcare quality and efficiency due to the creative use of health communication and health IT."[30]

Health communication as a public policy tool

There is long-standing interest in the role of health communication techniques and initiatives in advancing public health policy. Public health professionals can point to a number of communication and education campaigns that, over time, have had a demonstrable impact on public health goals. But the record is not universally positive, especially in the case of difficult public health challenges that disproportionately affect minorities and other underserved communities. As Hornik notes, "interventions which have relied primarily on communication and education have mostly failed to achieve substantial and sustainable results in terms of behavior change, and have made little impact in terms of closing the gap in health status between different social and economic groups in society."[19]

Still, policy makers continue to emphasize health communication as an integral element in efforts to advance public and population health goals, with particular interest in the promising technical tools available to amplify the impact of such initiatives.[31,32] This is noted explicitly by *Healthy People 2020*, which lists as one of its goals "[using] health communication strategies and health information technology (HIT) to improve population health outcomes and healthcare quality, and to achieve health equity."[30] The Institute of Medicine agreed as long ago as 2002 in its report *Speaking of Health,* which concluded that "communication interventions to affect health behavior are an increasingly important strategy for improving the health of the American people."[18] In particular, it noted that "the impressive growth of new communication technologies offers significant opportunities to integrate mass and micro communication strategies, allowing more effective and efficient population reach while permitting segmentation and even tailoring to diverse populations."[18]

Even with all the progress made since the Institute of Medicine's report was issued, the question of how best to leverage current and emerging communications technologies to most effectively support public health policy goals remains a complex one. *Healthy People 2020* acknowledges the challenge by noting the intricate mix of influencers at multiple levels—personal (biological, psychological); organizational and institutional; environmental (social and physical); and policy—that affect health and health behaviors. However, the dramatic advances in health communication and media technology and practice may offer public health professionals and policy makers their best hope of meeting that challenge.

Notes

1. History of Communication. History World website. http://www.historyworld .net/wrldhis/PlainTextHistories.asp?historyid=aa93.

2. Gascoigne B. History of Communication. 2001. History World website. http:// www.historyworld.net.

3. Manohar U. Why Is Communication Important? http://www.buzzle.com/ articles/why-is-communication-important.html.

4. Brecht M. *Martin Luther: His Road to Reformation 1483–1521.* Vol. 1. Trans. James L. Schaaf. Philadelphia: Fortress Press; 1985:204–205.

5. Hutchinson H. How the *Lancet* made medical history. BBC News. October 6, 2003. http://news.bbc.co.uk/2/hi/health/3168608.stm. Accessed December 7, 2011.

6. LeBrun J-L. *Scientific Writing: A Reader and Writer's Guide.* Hackensack, NJ: World Scientific; 2007.

7. The International DOI System. http://www.doi.org/.

8. Groves T. Sharing the raw data from medical research [corrected]. *BMJ.* 2009;338:b1285.

9. See www.nytimes.com/2012/04/17/science/rise-in-scientific-journal-retractions-prompts-calls-for-reform.html?pagewanted=all; Laine C, Goodman SN, Griswold ME, Sox HC. Reproducible research: Moving toward research the public can really trust. *Ann Intern Med.* 2007;146(6):450–453.

10. U.S. Department of Health and Human Services. *Healthy People 2010.* 2nd ed. Washington DC: U.S. Government Printing Office; 2000.

11. Cline R. American Public Health Association (APHA) Health Communication Working Group brochure. 2003. http://www.healthcommunication.net/APHA/APHA.html.

12. Schiavo R. *Health Communication: From Theory to Practice.* San Francisco: Jossey-Bass; 2007.

13. National Cancer Institute. *Making Health Communication Programs Work: A Planner's Guide.* Washington, DC: U.S. Government Printing Office; 2008.

14. Hornik R. Public health education and communication as policy instruments for bringing about changes in behavior. In: Goldberg M, Fishbein M, Middlestadt SE, eds. *Social Marketing: Theoretical and Practical Perspectives.* Mahwah, NJ: Lawrence Erlbaum Associates; 1997.

15. du Pré A. *Communicating about Health: Current Issues and Perspectives.* Mountain View, CA: Mayfield Press; 2000.

16. Maibach E, Parrott RL, eds. *Designing Health Messages: Approaches from Communication Theory and Public Health Practice.* Thousand Oaks, CA: Sage; 1995.

17. Thompson TL, Dorsey AM, Miller KI, Parrott R. *Handbook of Health Communication.* Mahwah, NJ: Lawrence Erlbaum Associates; 2003.

18. Committee on Communication for Behavior Change in the 21st Century, Institute of Medicine of the National Academies. *Speaking of Health: Assessing Health Communications Strategies for Diverse Populations.* Washington, DC: National Academies Press; 2002.

19. Hornik R. *Public Health Communication: Evidence for Behavior Change.* Mahwah, NJ: Lawrence Erlbaum Associates; 2002.

20. Maibach EW. Communication for health. *Encyclopedia of Public Health.* http://www.enotes.com/public-health-encyclopedia.

21. Siegel M, Doner L. *Marketing Public Health: Strategies to Promote Social Change.* Gaithersburg, MD: Aspen; 1998.

22. Noar SM. A 10-year retrospective of research in health mass media campaigns: Where do we go from here? *J Health Commun: Int Perspect.* 2006;11(1):21–42.

23. Kotler P, Roberto EL. *Social Marketing: Strategies for Changing Public Behavior.* New York: Free Press; 1989.

24. Northouse LL, Northouse PG. *Health Communication: Strategies for Health Professionals.* 3rd ed. Stamford, CT: Appleton and Lange; 1998.

25. Nutbeam D. Health literacy as a public health goal: A challenge for contemporary health education and communication strategies into the 21st century. *Health Promot Int.* 2000;15(3):259–267.

26. Shen Benjamin SP. Science literacy and the public understanding of science. In: Day S, ed. *Communication of Scientific Information.* Basel: Karger; 1975.

27. Neuhauser L, Kreps GL. Rethinking communication in the eHealth era. *J Health Psychol.* 2003;8(1):7–23.

28. Robinson TN, Patrick K, Eng TR, et al., for the Science Panel on Interactive Communication and Health. An evidence-based approach to interactive health communication: A challenge to medicine in the information age. *JAMA.* 1998;280:1264–1269.

29. Neuhauser L, Kreps GL. eHealth communication and behavior change: Promise and performance. *Soc Semiotics.* 2010;20(1):9–27.

30. U.S. Department of Health and Human Services. *Healthy People 2020.* http://www.healthypeople.gov/2020/.

31. Wallach L, Dorfman L. Media advocacy: A strategy for advancing policy and promoting health. *Health Educ Q.* 1996;23(3):293–317.

32. Calderon JL, Beltran RA. Pitfalls in health communication: Healthcare policy, institution, structure, and process. *Med Gen Med.* 2004;6(1):9.

Partnerships in Public Health

Working Together for a Mutual Benefit

Stephen W. Wyatt, Kevin T. Brady, and W. Ryan Maynard

For a clinician, providing comprehensive health care to an individual patient is complex and challenging, and it normally requires a wide variety of clinical disciplines over the individual's lifetime. The growth in clinical specialties and even subspecialties over the years, along with the development of an evolving cadre of support disciplines, demonstrates that ensuring the health of one patient has become a team effort. If caring for the health of an individual patient is this complex, imagine the issues associated with ensuring the health of a population—the mandate presented to public health practitioners and public health systems. This mandate encompasses a breadth of issues that would cause the weak-hearted to run—and to run quickly—from the challenge.

What challenges must public health address to keep the population healthy? They involve a range of issues, including environmental quality, restaurant inspections, disease surveillance, and disease prevention programs. The breadth and depth of these issues are quite daunting. Combine this with the reality that public health agencies and programs at the local, state, and federal levels are typically underfunded, understaffed, and underappreciated. This is a recipe for frustration, if not failure. Collaboration and partnerships are one potential solution to the scarcity of both human and fiscal resources. There is much to be done, resources are in short supply, and there are many critical opportunities that must be seized. This reality makes public health partnerships with business, education, and health care delivery systems a necessity, not a potential option to be considered. To disregard the need and the opportunity to partner could even be considered "malpractice."

The range of potential partners available to the public health practice community is not as limited as one might think. Several groups and types of organizations move to the top of the list as potential partners: voluntary health organizations, health-related foundations, health care delivery organizations, and companies or industries with health-related streams of business. Thinking broadly can expand this initial list significantly. For example, almost every business has a direct interest in improving the health of its workers. From there, it is not unreasonable to expand this interest to the health of the entire population in the company's geographic region and how the company impacts it. Today, with all the demands on public health, practitioners cannot be bound by conventional thinking and traditional public health partners; they must be creative. As the proverbial saying (often attributed to Plato) goes: necessity is the mother of invention.

For public health practice at the international, national, state, and local levels, this chapter explores the types of collaborations and potential partners available and provides examples and lessons learned from the published literature.

Partnership Types

Basically, there are two partnership types: informal and formal. Informal partnerships involve an exchange of information, endorsements, and ideas for actions that may lead to or evolve into more formal partnerships. Formal partnerships are typically characterized by the exchange of resources, expertise, dollars, staff time, branding, recognition, and so forth. Both types of partnerships may evolve into the next level of working relationship: collaborative agreements. The reasons for pursuing a partnership or a collaborative arrangement vary, but they often fall into several general areas: mutual benefit to the participating organizations, altruism, scientific advancement, or advancement of a specific health outcome.

Collaborative agreements can also be informal or formal. Informal collaborative agreements tend to be based on verbal or oral commitments, whereas formal collaborative agreements often take the form of grants or contracts and purchase orders to initiate the exchange of resources. Formal collaborative agreements generally define the parameters of the potential or agreed-on partnership, including the following: protection of interests, delineation of roles and responsibilities, limitations on other partners (e.g., not working with businesses with tobacco interests), time lines, authoritative assurances, scope of effort, and influence over a project or activity. There are four general types of collaborative agreements in public health practice settings:

1. Business agreements: Resources are normally fiscal and flow in one direction, from the business to the activity, with minimal input or representation from the business.

2. Foundation agreements: Resources typically flow in both directions (more give-and-take), but both parties operate within specific parameters.
3. Coalitions: These typically involve multiple partners; often include a complex exchange or sharing of resources and governance; and require the reporting and measurement of impact.
4. Contracts: These are typically detailed agreements that outline specific expectations of the partnership, its parameters, and the exchange of resources.

What Science Tells Us about Public Health Collaboration

With the foregoing definitions as context, a review of the published peer-reviewed literature on collaborations or partnerships in the public health practice setting produced interesting and informative examples. The selected articles cover a range of situations, including local collaborations, partnerships that target international or global public health issues and opportunities, and academic–public health practice partnerships.

A 2007 article by Buse and Harmer captures what the authors view as critical elements in successful global public health collaborations.[1] Their methodology included a qualitative assessment of global collaborations they were directly engaged in over a five-year period in the first decade of the twenty-first century. The authors also systematically reviewed the structure of more than 100 collaborative initiatives through an analysis of published literature, reports, and in-person interviews with individuals engaged in the collaborations. From this process, they developed lists of both effective and ineffective partnership habits. They identify the following as "healthy" habits:

- Commitment is required of all parties in the partnership, and conflicts of interest and divided loyalties must be addressed.
- Continuing review and oversight is required to maintain a healthy partnership.
- Collaborations must be adequately resourced to have an opportunity to succeed.
- Standard operating procedures should be adopted to improve both performance and accountability.
- The prevailing paradigm, which presupposes that market-based approaches are more efficient than public-sector ones, must be reassessed.
- Partnerships should strive for balanced representation of stakeholders on their governing or guiding bodies.

- Ownership, alignment, and harmonization with broader (in this case, international) planning and agendas are critical to ensure that the partnership fits with other efforts.

Buse and Harmer's list of effective habits evolved from their assessment of factors that resulted in less impact or a lack of overall success. They termed these the "unhealthy" habits:

- Alignment with other efforts is out of sync.
- Partnerships are not representative of their stakeholders.
- Governance or guidance is poor.
- Financial support is inadequate.
- There is poor harmonization.
- Incentives for partnership staff are inadequate.
- There is a diminished sense of the public nature of public health initiatives.

In a 2010 article, Coursey-Bailey focuses on the need to create partnerships across multiple sectors to impact the health of populations.[2] The article's introduction supports a concept noted in this chapter: "partnerships create a way forward when no clear solution exists and no single entity can claim the necessary expertise, authority or resources to bring about change." The author highlights several foundational elements or characteristics that are required to build and sustain successful partnerships: the social value of the effort, common goals among the collaborators, rewards or incentives, and comprehensive and coordinated approaches. Coursey-Bailey hypothesizes that partnerships make better use of existing resources and expand the range of potential partners to include faith-based organizations, businesses, and institutions involved in education, public safety, housing, and even transportation. The following actions are recommended to help build these important collaborative efforts:

- Establish metrics to both inform and motivate cross-sector action, with an emphasis on developing and including partnerships with the business community.
- Create opportunities for cross-sector networking and collaboration to build relationships between and among leaders.
- Adopt a network mind-set to overcome the seemingly intractable barriers to achieving success in improving the health of populations.
- Develop incentives for policy actions and leadership, while removing disincentives for participation.

- Develop and advocate for sustained, long-term funding mechanisms, as opposed to short-term support strategies (contracts and grants).
- Invest in data systems that allow the integration of multiple sources of data that can provide snapshots of the health and health improvement needs of populations and demonstrate impact after interventions.

Roussos and Fawcett provide a definition of public health partnerships: "collaborative partnerships attempt to improve conditions and outcomes related to the health and well being of entire communities."[3] They accurately note that these partnerships are often hybrid strategies that include aspects of social planning, community organizing, community development, and policy advocacy and may act as catalysts for community change. They argue that the distinguishing feature of such collaborative partnerships is broad community engagement in creating and sustaining conditions that promote behaviors associated with widespread health and well-being. They outline several notable obstacles to the successful organization and maintenance of effective partnerships:

- Confronting and overcoming conflict within the partnership and in the broader community.
- Maintaining adequate resources and continuity of leadership long enough to make a difference and see an impact.
- Engaging those in the community with the most experience related to the issue or concern.
- Sharing risks, resources, and responsibilities among participating individuals and organizations.
- Collaborating with community leaders in sectors outside the professional field of the lead organization in the partnership.

So far, the articles have provided a "macro-level" perspective on public health partnerships and collaborations. Another group of articles considers collaborations or partnerships between public health and business, health care, or academic institutions. A 2007 article by Curtis and colleagues is complementary and assesses opportunities and challenges specifically in the private sector.[4] The authors argue that the public sector typically brings political credibility or legitimacy, institutional anchors, a delivery infrastructure, access to resources and expertise, and a guiding vision to the table. They analyze a partnership between public health and business that addressed the promotion of hand washing to prevent the transmission of infectious disease. Through this partnership and the mass media interventions it developed, hand washing and hand soap sales increased, creating a win for both the public health and the business sectors and demonstrating that such collaborations are mutually beneficial.

A 2006 article by Buehler and colleagues examines the lessons learned from a specific emergency preparedness collaboration in Georgia, involving the distribution of medications from the strategic national stockpile.[5] This article also makes an interesting observation about surveys conducted by the National Business Group on Health (NBGH). Following the 2001 anthrax attacks, the NBGH surveyed selected large businesses and public health leaders on their attitudes about collaboration between the business and public health sectors. The findings were not surprising: respondents believed that collaboration and partnership opportunities were underdeveloped. However, the reasons given for this situation were a little more intriguing. Respondents cited inadequate or limited personal relationships between business and public health leaders and a lack of understanding of their respective capabilities and vulnerabilities. Business and public health leaders also mentioned the lack of familiarity with each other's values, metrics, and resources; differences in terminology; and variations in modes of operation. Further, both public health practitioners and businesspeople battled the stereotypical views or perspectives of their counterparts. For example, public health practitioners were suspicious of the profit motives of individuals from the business sector, whereas businesspeople viewed public servants as inefficient and wasteful. The finding that personal relationships are potentially important for the development of partnership opportunities may be surprising at first. But after reflecting on this finding, it becomes much less surprising because in many cultures, business decisions (and creating a partnership is a strategic business decision) are based on either established or yet to be developed relationships.

In a 2000 article, Halverson and colleagues explore factors that influence collaborations and partnerships between the public health and health care (medical) sectors.[6] They conducted a telephone survey of sixty county public health directors in the United States regarding their relationships with community health centers and community hospitals. Consistent with findings from other studies, the authors found that the decision to collaborate is influenced by or contingent on the underlying institutional missions. Results from the study indicated that 55 percent of the hospitals and 64 percent of the community health centers were engaged in active collaboration with the public health sector. Public hospitals were more than twice as likely as private, nonprofit hospitals to participate in collaborative relationships. Further, for-profit hospitals were less than half as likely to collaborate as nonprofit hospitals. It was not surprising that most of the collaborative relationships focused on patient care or patient referral agreements and that less than 40 percent were formal agreements.

Partnerships and collaborations between institutions of higher education, both public and private, and the public health sector at the local, state, and national levels are fairly common. Numerous federal public health agencies in the United States, including the National Institutes of Health, Centers for Disease Control and Prevention (CDC), and Health Resources and Services Administration, have well-established, long-term partnerships with academic institutions. These partnerships typically involve financial support for basic, applied, and translational research by faculty members at the academic institutions. These agencies also support faculty and their institutions in more applied public health efforts, ranging from disease surveillance to training for the state and local public health workforce. The development of cancer registries in academic institutions—first as part of the National Cancer Institute's Surveillance, Epidemiology, and End Results Program and later as an integral component of the CDC's National Program of Cancer Registries—is illustrative. Although most state cancer registries were developed and are guided by state public health agencies, academic institutions have added significant value to this national public health surveillance network. In addition to the fiscal relationships between academics (and their institutions) and federal public health organizations, faculty members are valuable resources for advisory committees, review panels, and other entities in the federal public health sector.

The depth and breadth of relationships between state public health agencies and academic institutions vary significantly across the country. Arguably, a snapshot of the partnerships and collaborations that exist today would look quite different from one taken months or years from now. Obviously, these relationships, partnerships, and collaborations change over time. Shifts in the leadership of state government are one reason for change. For example, one administration may focus on downsizing state government—a popular theme—and outsourcing critical activities to a variety of sources, including academic institutions and their faculty and staff. With such outsourcing, the size of the state workforce is often reduced, resulting in a reduced capacity at the state public health agency. For the organization that receives the outsourced work, fiscal resources accrue, along with a set of expectations and opportunities for increased interaction between the state public health agency and its staff. However, a new administration in the state government may result in a rapid reversal. Efforts to rebuild core capacity at the state government level may occur, based on the belief that outsourcing or contracting with an academic institution for capacity or infrastructure is more expensive than building it internally.

In a 2007 article, Livingood and colleagues[7] note the emphasis on collaboration between academic institutions and public health organizations contained in both the 1988 and 2003 reports by the Institute of Medicine.[8, 9] The 1988 report highlights the perspective that "schools of public health had become rather isolated from the field of public health practice." Keck credits the "academic health department" concept for reinvigorating the interest in collaboration between public health and academic institutions.[10] Other investigators have compared this public health practice–academic center collaboration to the well-established collaborations between teaching hospitals and medical schools within academic medical centers.[11, 12]

The Livingood research was a mixed-method study of sixty-seven county health department directors and administrators in Florida, yielding a response rate of 76 percent. The study included in-person interviews as well as archived data and information to provide context for potential partnerships. The research explored the quantitative aspects of academic–public health collaboration in Florida, as well as qualitative perspectives such as the types of collaboration and the associated problems, challenges, and recommendations. The authors found that 82 percent of the surveyed county health departments had formal, established relationships with academic institutions covering a broad range of partnership efforts that supported capacity building, education, health services, and research (including evaluation). The following recommendations for advancing collaboration between academic institutions and local health departments emerged from this study:

- Develop a recognition process (i.e., a review and approval process similar to the accreditation process) for academic health departments as a mechanism for creating awareness of and support for collaboration with academic institutions.
- Explore and better define the academic-agency relationship and what both institutions can gain from the effort.
- Develop recommendations and guidelines for memoranda of agreement and contracts between agencies and academic institutions.
- Design model legislation for local and state governments to sustain and expand partnerships.
- Encourage state health departments to leverage their influence with the legislature, university, and community college systems and with sister departments to facilitate and support the development of local academic health departments.

New Ways to Collaborate

At a recent congressional briefing on Capitol Hill regarding hepatitis prevention and treatment, the assistant secretary for health, Howard K. Koh, reinforced a sentiment often expressed by government officials: government cannot do it alone. He referenced a coalition of outside businesses that supports the CDC's efforts to control hepatitis and is managed through the CDC Foundation—an example of an innovative approach to further public health activities that involves multiple partners. In addition to the CDC, the National Institutes of Health, the Department of Defense, and the National Parks Service have their own nonprofit foundations. Similarly, state health departments (e.g., North Carolina) and city health departments (e.g., New York City) have established these types of organizations to assist with their mission. All recognize the value of a separate entity that can form partnerships outside of traditional government funding mechanisms.

As an example, the CDC Foundation was established as an independent, nonprofit 501(c)(3) organization to forge effective partnerships between the CDC and other entities to further the agency's mission. As the foundation states on its website: "The CDC Foundation helps CDC pursue innovative ideas that need support from outside partners. The support needed is most often funding, but also can include expertise, information, leadership or connections to specific groups of people. CDC Foundation partnerships help CDC launch new programs, expand existing programs that show promise, or establish a proof of concept through a pilot project before scaling it up. In each partnership, outside support gives CDC experts the flexibility to quickly and effectively connect with the right partners, information and technology needed to address a priority public health challenge." In return, partners (businesses, philanthropies, and organizations) help expand important public health initiatives that align with their missions and their work, gain access to mutually beneficial collaborations with world-renowned CDC scientists, and enjoy the advantages of a simplified process of partnering with a complex federal agency.

The CDC Foundation has established the following characteristics of collaborative partner activities to ensure effective collaboration and transparency with outside businesses:

- Well-defined and substantial public health benefit based on sound science and the public good
- Clear, identifiable, substantial leadership role for CDC and a designated lead and champion within the agency

- Ideas that have been reviewed and approved by CDC's Office of the Director
- Activities with a manageable size and scope with specific time lines and milestones
- Funding that is not revocable or contingent on any action by CDC other than actions described in the proposal documents (including, for example, the official results of a symposium, the participation of certain individuals in the event, etc.)
- Non-exclusivity in the proposed activity meaning other partners may join at any time
- Outcomes of the activity are not intended for direct monetary benefit for the partner; avoidance of conflicts of interest
- Adherence to the requirements for independence and objectivity of scientific judgment as set forth in CDC's "Guidelines for Collaboration with the Private Sector"
- Deference to CDC's final judgment on all matters of scientific findings, facts or recommendations
- Equal access to results of findings for the public and partners
- Demonstrate opportunities for return on investment for public health, CDC, the CDC Foundation and its partners

The foundation further states that it will not support partnerships in which there is no clear mission compatibility or that ask for product endorsements. CDC co-branding is allowed only if the official CDC review committee approves it for this purpose. Since 1995, the CDC Foundation has provided more than $300 million to support projects with the CDC.

The process of funding projects through the CDC Foundation usually begins when a scientist or program expert at the CDC has an idea to expand a specific public health activity but recognizes that the agency lacks the resources to fund the effort. CDC employees often have the opportunity to discuss their public health projects at professional meetings that may be attended by representatives of potential donors. If one of these representatives recognizes that the employee's project matches the donor organization's philanthropic mission, the CDC Foundation is engaged to secure agreements and put in place the necessary firewalls to protect the science developed by the CDC. Once a concept is approved and agreements are in place, the donor's resources can be used in a variety of creative ways, such as securing research fellows or consultants, expediting contracts for specialized services or fieldwork, purchasing equipment and supplies, and facilitating travel for the CDC team and other project partners. Given that the CDC Foundation manages approximately 200 projects, it is clear that many organizations recognize the value of such partnerships. The foundation raised more than $40 million for the CDC during 2010—a good indication that outside businesses are eager to work with this federal agency.

Closing Perspectives

Any business or organization that is not focused on thriving in its particular fiscal or cultural environment is an entity that is in decline. For an organization to thrive in and respond to the current environment, flexibility and creativity are a necessity—and the more challenging the environment, the more important they become. Without such a perspective, businesses and organizations may die. These basic perspectives on surviving and thriving apply to public health organizations and entities as much as they do to Fortune 500 companies. Even in the most positive fiscal and policy environments, public health is challenged to grow and expand. The sad fact is that most opportunities for expansion evolve from major health challenges or threats. Once the threat has apparently disappeared or dissipated, support for the public health effort and infrastructure often diminishes. Although this may change in the future, such a perspective is risky. It is dangerous not to plan for and pursue different paradigms to position public health to meet future challenges and opportunities. Expanding the universe of potential partners and collaborators makes both practical and business sense. Depending on the government alone to improve and protect the health of the public is naïve at best. The challenges to public health are likely to become increasingly complex and difficult. Recognizing that these challenges will likely require both new and enhanced resources is critical, as is the effort to partner with both traditional and new and evolving organizations and to create collaborations that will effectively position public health for the future.

Notes

1. Buse K, Harmer AM. Seven habits of highly effective global public-private health partnerships: Practice and potential. *Soc Sci Med.* 2007;64:259–271.

2. Coursey-Bailey SB. Focusing on solid partnerships across multiple sectors for population health improvement. *Preventing Chronic Dis.* 2010;7(6):1–3.

3. Roussos ST, Fawcett SB. A review of collaborative partnerships as a strategy for improving community health. *Annu Rev Public Health.* 2000;21:369–402.

4. Curtis VA, Garbrah-Aidoo N, Scott B. Masters of marketing: Bringing private sector skills to public health partnerships. *Am J Public Health.* 2007;97(4):634–641.

5. Buehler JW, Whitney EA, Berkelman RL. Business and public health

collaboration for emergency preparedness in Georgia: A case study. *BMC Public Health.* 2006;6:285. http://www.biomedcentral.com/1471–2458/6/285.

6. Halverson PK, Mays GP, Kaluzny AD. Working together? Organizational and market determinants of collaboration between public health and medical care providers. *Am J Public Health.* 2000;90(12):1913–1916.

7. Livingood WC, Goldhagen J, Little W, Gornto J, Hou T. Assessing the status of partnerships between academic institutions and public health agencies. *Am J Public Health.* 2007;97:659–666.

8. Institute of Medicine. *The Future of Public Health.* Washington, DC: National Academies Press; 1988.

9. Institute of Medicine. *Who Will Keep the Public Healthy? Educating Public Health Professionals for the 21st Century.* Washington, DC: National Academies Press; 2003.

10. Keck CW. Lessons learned from an academic health department. *J Public Health Manage Pract.* 2000;6(1):47–52.

11. Meyer D, Armstrong-Coben A, Batista M. How a community-based organization and an academic health center are creating an effective partnership for training and service. *Acad Med.* 2005;80(4):327–333.

12. Naughton J, Vana JE. The academic health center and the healthy community. *Am J Public Health.* 1994;84(7):1071–1076.

10

The Organizational Landscape of the American Public Health System

Paul K. Halverson, Glen P. Mays, and Rachel Hogg

Public health is practiced in the United States through the collective actions of governmental and private organizations that vary widely in their resources, missions, and operations.[1-3] Governmental public health agencies play central roles in these delivery systems, but most of them rely heavily on their ability to inform, influence, communicate, and collaborate with numerous external organizations that contribute to public health services.[4] The range of organizations involved in public health delivery and the division of responsibility between governmental and private organizations vary widely across communities.[5-7] Within the governmental sector, public health agencies differ in their statutorily defined powers and duties and in the extent to which these powers are exercised at the state level versus delegated to the local level.[8]

The complexity of the interorganizational and intergovernmental structure poses a challenge to understanding the full extent of the public health enterprise in the United States and to identifying policy and management strategies to improve its performance. This chapter describes the American public health system in a way that highlights the organizational contributors to governmental public health services, as well as those organizations and individuals that contribute to public health at the community level. Understanding how public health services are delivered and the complex nature of the system's interdependence will allow a better understanding of public health as it is practiced in America today.

Conceptualizing the Public Health System

To understand the totality of the American public health system, an operational definition is required that delineates public health's scope of activity and the range of actors participating in the system. Although much has been written about public health, perhaps the most cited source for action in public health policy is the 1988 report of the Institute of Medicine (IOM). In *The Future of Public Health,* the IOM describes the mission of public health as "fulfilling society's interest in assuring conditions in which people can be healthy." It further defines the role of public health agencies at all levels of government as "assessment, policy development, and assurance."[9]

Many worthwhile studies have been conducted since the IOM published this landmark work, but no organization, including subsequent IOM panels, has better defined public health, and no one has questioned the report's primary findings. After a careful consideration of the facts, the IOM declared the American public health system to be in "disarray."[9] A revealing characterization of this system appears in the concluding remarks: "This report conveys an urgent message to the American people. Public health is a vital function that is in trouble. Immediate public concern and support are called for in order to fulfill society's interest in assuring the conditions in which people can be healthy. History teaches us that an organized community effort to prevent disease and promote health is both valuable and effective. Yet public health in the United States has been taken for granted, and public health responsibilities have become so fragmented that deliberate action is often difficult if not impossible."[9] Since a vibrant and effective public health system is so important to the success of the American health system, ensuring a better understanding of public health and the benefits of an effective public health system becomes an important task not only for students of public health but also for any conscientious citizen who engages in constructive discourse about improving the health of Americans and reforming the health care system.

Many people outside the public health profession perceive that the public health system functions primarily to provide health care to the poor and disadvantaged at publicly owned and operated clinics or hospitals. Some recognize public health's role in the administration of childhood immunizations at public clinics or schools, and others associate public health with the testing of drinking water and wells or the inspection of restaurants. Most people would be surprised to learn the many different services, functions, and issues that public health undertakes to ensure, in the IOM's words, "the circumstances in which people can be healthy."[9]

Part of the reason for the confusion is the wide variety of services performed by public health organizations. Although public health services may include the provision of medical care, particularly in southern states, the IOM framework provides for a much broader role than is currently understood by most of the public. The IOM defines the three core functions of public health as follows:

Assessment: The committee recommends that every public health agency regularly and systematically collect, assemble, analyze, and make available information on the health of the community, including statistics on health status, community health needs, and epidemiologic and other studies of health problems.

Policy Development: The committee recommends that every public health agency exercise its responsibility to serve the public interest in the development of comprehensive public health policies by promoting use of the scientific knowledge base in decision-making about public health and by leading in developing public health policy. Agencies must take a strategic approach, developed on the basis of a positive appreciation for the democratic political process.

Assurance: The committee recommends that public health agencies assure their constituents that services necessary to achieve agreed upon goals are provided, either by encouraging actions by other entities (private or public sector), by requiring such action through regulation, or by providing services directly. The committee recommends that each public health agency involve key policymakers and the general public in determining a set of high-priority personal and community-wide health services that governments will guarantee to every member of the community. This guarantee should include subsidization or direct provision of high-priority personal health services for those unable to afford them.[9]

Following the IOM report, the U.S. Department of Health and Human Services established a working group within the Office of Disease Prevention and Health Promotion to further specify and refine the public health system's vision, mission, and roles (see box). The Public Health Functions Steering Committee devised a consensus statement that has become widely used to characterize contemporary public health practice. This statement defines both the core functions and the essential services of public health, and it has become one of the most frequently used illustrations of how key activities support the central mission of public health in operational terms (table 10.1). The essential services defined in the consensus statement have been used to establish performance expectations and standards for public health agencies and systems and to develop measures to track and improve their work. For example, standards and measures based on these essential services have become central components of the National Public Health Performance Standards Program of the Centers for Disease Control and Prevention (CDC; see www.cdc.gov/

Public Health Vision, Mission, and Roles

Vision: Healthy people in healthy communities

Mission: Promote physical and mental health and prevent disease, injury, and disability

Public health:

- Prevents epidemics and the spread of disease
- Protects against environmental hazards
- Prevents injuries
- Promotes and encourages healthy behaviors
- Responds to disasters and assists communities in recovery
- Assures the quality and accessibility of health services

Essential public health services:

- Monitor health status to identify community health problems
- Diagnose and investigate health problems and health hazards in the community
- Inform, educate, and empower people about health issues
- Mobilize community partnerships to identify and solve health problems
- Develop policies and plans that support individual and community health efforts
- Enforce laws and regulations that protect health and ensure safety
- Link people to needed personal health services and assure the provision of health care
- Assure a competent public health and personal health care workforce
- Evaluate effectiveness, accessibility, and quality of personal and population-based health services
- Research for new insights and innovative solutions to health problems

Source: Public Health Functions Steering Committee. Public Health in America. 2005. http://www.health.gov/phfunctions/public.htm.

NPHPSP) and, more recently, of the national public health agency accreditation program developed by the Public Health Accreditation Board (PHAB).

Identifying "Systemness" in Public Health

A public health system comprises "all public, private, and voluntary entities that contribute to the delivery of essential public health services within

Table 10.1. Core Functions and Essential Services in Public Health			
Assessment	Monitor health	System management	Research
	Diagnose and investigate		
Policy development	Inform, educate, empower		
	Mobilize community partnerships		
	Develop policies		
Assurance	Enforce laws		
	Link to/provide care		
	Assure competent workforce		
	Evaluate		

Source: Public Health Functions Steering Committee. July 1995.

a jurisdiction."[10] In other words, a public health system is a network of actors with differing roles, relationships, and interactions that influence the health of a defined population. All these entities contribute to the health and well-being of the population by virtue of what they do and how they interact. Governmental public health agencies, at both state and local levels, are leading players in public health systems, but these agencies rarely if ever provide the full spectrum of essential public health services for a state or community. Hospitals, public safety agencies, voluntary health organizations, mental health centers, schools, civic groups, faith institutions, and many others contribute to accomplishing the actions necessary to achieve public health. Some of the most frequent and intensive actors within the system include the following:

- Health care providers such as hospitals, physicians, community health centers, mental health facilities, laboratories, nursing homes, and others that provide preventive, curative, and rehabilitative care.
- Public safety agencies such as police, fire, and emergency medical services (EMS), whose work is focused on preventing and coping with injury and other emergency health situations.
- Human service and charitable organizations such as food banks, public assistance agencies, transportation providers, and others that assist people in gaining access to health care and other health-enhancing services.
- Educational and youth development organizations such as schools, faith institutions, youth centers, and others groups that help to inform, educate, and prepare children so they can make informed decisions and act responsibly regarding health and other life choices.
- Recreation and arts-related organizations that contribute to the physical

and mental well-being of the community and those that live, work, and play in it.
- Economic and philanthropic organizations such as employers, community development and zoning boards, United Way, and community and business foundations that provide resources necessary for individuals and organizations to survive and thrive in the community.

State Public Health Agencies

Public health agencies exist at all levels of the government: federal, state, and local. In addition, public health services are provided within the context of the governmental authority in both tribal and territorial settings. Although the concepts of a public health system emphasize that multiple contributors are required to deliver public health services effectively, the primary orchestration point for most systems rests with governmental public health agencies, particularly those at the state level.

The U.S. government was founded on a set of principles established in the Constitution that reserves all powers not specifically granted to the federal government to the states. Although health matters are increasingly debated at the national level, very few health-related powers are explicitly delegated to the federal government. Generally, the federal government's role in public health, aside from specific matters of interstate commerce and in national emergencies, is limited to taxation and spending on public health programs (federal public health agencies are covered in more detail later). This legal framework establishes that the primary public health jurisdiction is assigned to the government within the sovereign borders of each state. The issue of sovereignty may seem like an artifact to the casual reader, but it is the fundamental basis for the marked variation in states' organization, funding, and delivery of public health services. This state-by-state organization of public health systems also explains the variations among local public health jurisdictions. Whether they are counties, cities, or combinations of local jurisdictions, they are established by the laws of each state. The relationship between the state and its local units of government is shaped by the constitutional grant of authority and responsibility and by the laws, customs, and practices established among the governmental entities in each state or commonwealth.

The IOM recommends the following core public health responsibilities and authorities for state governments:

- The committee believes that states are and must be the central force in public health. They bear primary public sector responsibility for health.

- The committee recommends that the public health duties of states should include the following:

  - Assessment of health needs in the state based on statewide data collection;
  - Assurance of an adequate statutory base for health activities in the state;
  - Establishment of statewide health objectives, delegating power to localities as appropriate and holding them accountable;
  - Assurance of appropriate organized statewide effort to develop and maintain essential personal, educational, and environmental health services; provision of access to necessary services; and solution of problems inimical to health;
  - Guarantee of a minimum set of essential health services; and
  - Support of local service capacity, especially when disparities in local ability to raise revenue and/or direct action by the state to achieve adequate service levels.[9]

Although the states have made notable efforts to adopt uniform public health responsibilities such as those articulated by the IOM, state governmental health agencies vary widely in their powers and activities. Core responsibilities held by the vast majority of state health agencies include the following:

- Implementing effective statewide prevention programs such as tobacco quit lines, newborn screening programs, and disease surveillance.
- Assuring a basic level of community public health services across the state, regardless of the resources or capacities of local health departments.
- Engaging the services of professionals with specialized skills, such as disease outbreak specialists and restaurant and food services inspectors, who bring expertise that is hard to find, is too expensive to employ at the local level, or involves overseeing local public health functions.
- Collecting and analyzing statewide vital statistics, health indicators, and morbidity data to target public health threats and diseases, such as cancer.
- Investigating disease outbreaks, environmental hazards such as chemical spills, and other public health emergencies.
- Monitoring funds and other resources to ensure that they are used effectively and equitably throughout the state.
- Conducting statewide health planning, improvement, and evaluation.
- Licensing and regulating health care, food services, and other facilities.

There are some notable variations in state public health authority and responsibilities. For example, a slight majority (55 percent) of state public health agencies are structured as freestanding agencies, while the remaining 45 percent are located within an umbrella agency of state government. In thirteen states and the District of Columbia (28 percent), local health services are provided by the state public health agency (centralized, with no local health departments). In nineteen states (37 percent), local health services are provided by independent local health departments (decentralized). The remaining eighteen states (35 percent) function with some combination of these arrangements (hybrid). Seventy-two percent of state health agencies planned to seek accreditation through a voluntary national accreditation program; of those, 47 percent planned to seek accreditation within the first two years of the accreditation program (2011–2012). More than 40 percent of state public health agencies operate with fewer than 1,000 full-time employees (or the equivalent); less than 10 percent, however, have more than 5,000 full-time equivalents (the median is 1,224).[11]

State health agency organization and function

The organizational structure of state health agencies varies widely across the United States. The distinction between independent state health agencies and umbrella agencies is a defining feature, with considerable political, economic, and administrative implications. Umbrella agencies encompass a mix of administrative components and functions. Of the twenty-three states where the state health department operates within a larger umbrella agency or superagency, about 83 percent reported that the agency included the state's Medicaid program, and almost 80 percent claimed that the state public assistance program was a component of the agency.[11]

Placement of the state health department within an umbrella agency or superagency of the state government is a frequent source of contention among both policy makers and health policy experts. Some policy makers assert that costs decrease when health and health-related agencies are combined in one superagency, but there is no clear evidence that real and sustainable savings occur. The IOM's 1988 report, *The Future of Public Health*, examined the issue of umbrella agencies in state government and recommended that "each state have a department of health that groups all primarily health-related functions under professional direction—separate from income maintenance."[9] Further, the committee suggested "that the director of the department of health be a cabinet (or equivalent) officer. Ideally, the director should have doctoral-level education as a physician or in another health profession, as well as education in public health itself and extensive public sector administrative experience."[9] Although several states have created umbrella agencies since the report was issued, others have decided to reestablish separate state health departments. No conclusive research has been conducted that supports the cost-effectiveness of the economy-of-scale argument, and several state health officials have reported significant disadvantages in being combined with other agencies.

The most frequent concerns raised by state health officials include loss of a direct link to the governor and the legislature to communicate about health policy and health information; increased bureaucracy within the umbrella agency that does not fit the state health department's unique requirements for personnel, information systems, and procurement; decreased timeliness in responding to health needs and requirements due to more complex reporting and the filtering effects of indirect communication; and the general loss of focus on public health (sometimes accompanied by a loss of budget) in favor of the public financing of medical care. The barriers to a serious and objective analysis of the umbrella agency issue are significant because of the political and often partisan context in which these organizational decisions are made.

The relationship between the state health department and local public health agencies is another important organizational component. Data from the 2007 Association of State and Territorial Health Officials (ASTHO) *Chartbook of Public Health* demonstrated that roughly 8 percent of the states have no local health departments, and 55 percent operate either centralized or hybrid organizations;[12] these numbers remained the same in the 2010 ASTHO profile.[11] In a centralized organization, the local health agency is generally considered an administrative unit of the state government that is operated at the local level (usually the county); most (if not all) of the public health employees working at the local level are state employees. Funding operates through a state health department appropriations process. In a decentralized model, the local health agencies are autonomous units of local government (usually the county), the public health employees are local government employees, and funding flows through the local government entity. In a hybrid model, autonomous locally controlled and sponsored health agencies may exist in conjunction with state-controlled and -financed health agencies. In many cases, larger jurisdictions choose to fund and operate their own health department, whereas smaller jurisdictions may be served by a state-funded and -operated local health agency. In some small or less populated states, the state may choose not to operate any local health agencies at all. Elsewhere, the state or groups of local jurisdictions may operate regional health departments. The organization and financing of local health agencies can be a subject of heated debate between policy makers and directors of state and local health departments. Although some research has been conducted to better understand the effectiveness of various organizational models,[13] there is a clear need for additional and more comprehensive studies to guide decision makers.

State health agency priorities and activities

State health agencies also vary in how they conduct the functions and services for which they are responsible under state law. While all state health agencies have an epidemiologic function, including responsibility for investigating and controlling communicable diseases, 73 percent reported being responsible for rural health issues, and 51 percent were responsible for organizing and coordinating EMS. Forty-two state health agencies regulate hospitals directly or by contract; some also have responsibility for food processing regulation. About 24 percent of state health agencies are responsible for the licensure of nurses and physicians, and 22 percent for dentists. Roughly 22 percent of state health agencies administer the state medical examiner's office (for the full list of state health department functions and responsibilities, see the ASTHO's 2010 profile at www.ASTHO.org). At least 90 percent of state health agencies provide the following functions directly:

- Adult and child vaccine order management and inventory distribution.
- Maintenance of childhood immunization registry.
- Laboratory testing for bioterrorism agents, food-borne illnesses, and influenza typing.
- Data collection and analysis.
- Maintenance of vital records, as well as data on morbidity and reportable diseases.
- Epidemiology and surveillance activities for injuries, chronic diseases, and communicable diseases.
- Tracking of perinatal events or risk factors.
- Tobacco control and prevention.
- Food safety education.
- Preparedness.[11]

A topic of frequent discussion and debate is state health departments' and local public health agencies' direct provision of clinical services. The range of clinical services delivered by public health agencies varies from preventive services to obstetrical care and general primary care services. In Arkansas, for example, over two-thirds of all childhood immunizations are provided by staff of the state health agency. In addition, the Arkansas state health agency, which directly operates the county health departments, provides prenatal care, a full range of family planning services, and communicable disease diagnosis and treatment (including sexually transmitted diseases, tuberculosis diagnosis, and directly observed therapy). Public health agencies in Arkansas and Alabama are also major providers of home care services. Public health clinics in Tennessee and Florida include those classified as federally qualified community health centers, which provide a full range of primary care services (and, in some cases, dental services) on-site. Many southern states have a long history and experience in providing direct clinical services through public health agencies. In other parts of the United States, state and local public health agencies play more limited roles in the delivery of clinical services. Some public health policy experts criticize the distraction caused by the delivery of services to individual patients and the conflict created when an agency acts as both a provider and a regulator of services. Others cite the importance of public health agencies as providers of services to those who have nowhere else to turn.

Perhaps even more important than the full range of services provided by state health departments is their prioritizing of services and functions based on the needs of the state. This is especially true in the current environment of reduced investment in public health and pressure for budget cuts in state health departments. Given the IOM's recommendations related to supporting local public health services, it is reassuring to see that in a 2010 survey of state health officials, their most frequently listed priority was "infrastructure/capacity/IT [information technology]/workforce," followed by "quality improvement" (table 10.2).[11] In contrast, respondents to a 2007 survey listed disease prevention (45.5 percent), emergency preparedness (34 percent), and epidemiology, surveillance,

Table 10.2. Top Priorities Identified by State and Territorial Health Officials, 2010		
Priority	Number of Mentions	Percentage of Respondents
Infrastructure/capacity/IT/workforce	40	17
Quality improvement	21	9
Health promotion/prevention	18	8
Obesity, nutrition, and physical activity	14	6
Emergency preparedness	14	6
Health care reform	13	5
Communicable disease control	13	5
Environmental health	11	5
Tobacco	10	4
Strategic planning	10	4
Disparities	10	4
Chronic disease control	10	4
Funding and mitigating cuts	10	4
Other priorities	37	19

Source: Association of State and Territorial Health Officials. *Profile of State Public Health*. Vol. 2. Washington, DC: ASTHO; 2011.

and monitoring (31.8 percent) as the top three priorities.[12] Note that prepared-ness fell from the second to the fifth spot. However, it is important to note that if this survey had been conducted fifteen years ago, it is doubtful that prepared-ness would have made even the top ten priorities of most state health officials. But since the tragic events of 9/11 and the anthrax scares that followed, there has been an appropriate national focus on "all hazards" preparedness, given the im-portance of health in nearly all aspects of homeland defense, and public health has gained much higher visibility at all levels of government.

State public health financing

In many ways, state health department activities correlate strongly with the origin of their funding, and financing is an important topic of discussion in any description of state public health agencies. Public health finance has tak-en several twists and turns over the past decades, and although gathering fi-nancial information is simplistic in concept, it is quite complex in practice. One difficulty in collecting financial data is the realization that unlike most other public sectors, public health does not have a uniform chart of accounts to define data elements that can then be used for comparative reporting. Over the last few years, research in public health financing has expanded, with projects designed to examine the causes and consequences of variations in public health expenditures across states and communities and the returns to be gained from investments in public health.[14-18]

State health agencies access an array of funding sources to support their operations. On average, the largest funder of state public health is the federal government (46 percent), followed by state general revenue in a distant second place (22 percent). Other state and territorial funds generally include those from the tobacco master settlement agreement, as well as other designated or restricted funds, and together they equate to roughly 16 percent of state rev-enue.[19] Determining state health departments' revenue sources provides im-portant insight into why they pay such close attention to changes in federal funding and priorities.

State health agencies have had to absorb substantial funding reductions in recent years as a result of the economic downturn in 2007 and the subsequent shortfall in tax collection at the state level. Different from cuts in the past de-cade, the more recent cuts involve program elimination and staff layoffs that have drastically reduced the capacity of many state health departments (figure 10.1). Although it can be challenging to build new programs and expand im-portant initiatives that will make a substantial difference in the public's health, it is even more difficult to lay off employees or cut programs.

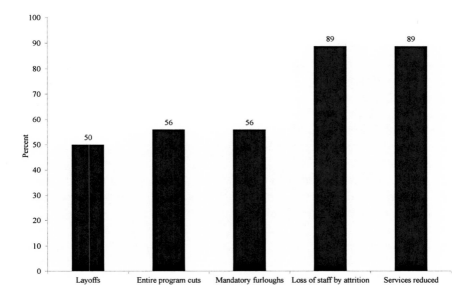

Figure 10.1. Percentage of state health agencies reporting selected responses to the economic recession, 2008–2010. *Source:* Association of State and Territorial Health Officials. *Budget Cuts Continue to Affect the Health of Americans: Update May 2011.* Washington, DC: ASTHO; 2011.

State public health workforce

The state public health workforce generally reflects the size of the jurisdiction and the range of services offered by the state health department. Obviously, states with a centralized local public health system have more personnel than those using a decentralized or hybrid model of service delivery and thereby relying more heavily on local government workers. The number of programs and regulatory functions assigned to the state health department can also impact workforce size. Workers fall into various classifications, including full-time equivalents, part-time, contractual, and hourly or temporary employees. The majority of state health agencies reported having fewer than 1,000 full-time equivalents.[11]

Local Public Health Agencies

States, territories, and tribes delegate certain public health powers and duties to local public health agencies, as specified in their constitutions, statutes, and regulations. Counties, cities, or towns are often designated local public health jurisdictions. The National Association of County and City Health Officials (NACCHO) defines a local public health agency as "an administrative or service unit of local or state government, concerned with health, and carrying some responsibility for the health of a jurisdiction smaller than the state."[20] Although their scope of activity varies widely across communities, local public health agencies typically shoulder the bulk of the responsibility for implementing public health programs within the community and delivering public health services, along with selected duties to enforce public health laws and regulations.

NACCHO has also created an operational definition that describes what every citizen should expect from a local public health agency. According to NACCHO, a functional local health department is one that:

- Elucidates the specific health issues confronting the community and how physical, behavioral, environmental, social, and economic conditions affect them.
- Investigates health problems and health threats.
- Prevents, minimizes, and contains adverse health effects from communicable diseases, disease outbreaks from unsafe food and water, chronic diseases, environmental hazards, injuries, and risky health behaviors.
- Leads planning and response activities for public health emergencies.
- Collaborates with other local responders and with state and federal agencies to intervene in other emergencies with public health significance (e.g., natural disasters).
- Implements health promotion programs.
- Engages the community to address public health issues.
- Develops partnerships with public and private health care providers and institutions, community-based organizations, and other government agencies (e.g., housing authority, criminal justice, education) engaged in services that affect health to collectively identify, alleviate, and act on the sources of public health problems.
- Coordinates the public health system's efforts in an intentional, noncompetitive, and nonduplicative manner.
- Addresses health disparities.
- Serves as an essential resource for local governing bodies and policy makers on up-to-date public health laws and policies.
- Provides science-based, timely, and culturally competent health information and health alerts to the media and to the community.

- Provides its expertise to others who treat or address issues of public health significance.
- Ensures compliance with public health laws and ordinances, using enforcement authority when appropriate.
- Employs well-trained staff members who have the necessary resources to implement best practices and evidence-based programs and interventions.
- Facilitates research efforts, when approached by researchers, that benefit the community.
- Uses and contributes to the evidence base of public health.
- Strategically plans its services and activities, evaluates performance and outcomes, and makes adjustments as needed to continually improve its effectiveness, enhance the community's health status, and meet the community's expectations.[20]

The IOM also developed specific recommendations about the powers and duties of local public health agencies, including the following:

- Assessment, monitoring, and surveillance of local health problems and needs and of resources for dealing with them.
- Policy development and leadership that foster local involvement and a sense of ownership, that emphasize local needs, and that advocate the equitable distribution of public resources and complementary private activities commensurate with community health needs.
- Assurance that high-quality services, including personal health services, needed for the protection of public health in the community are available and accessible to all persons; that the community receives proper consideration in the allocation of federal and state as well as local resources for public health; and that the community is informed about how to obtain public health, including personal health services, or how to comply with public health requirements.[9]

Local public health agencies (which number nearly 2,900 nationwide) vary widely in their organizational structure and governance. Key elements of this structural variation include the following: Sixty-eight percent of agencies served a county or combined city-county jurisdiction. Sixty-three percent served small jurisdictions (populations of less than 50,000), but these small jurisdictions accounted for only 1 percent of the U.S. population. The largest 5 percent of agencies served 49 percent of the U.S. population. Seventy-five percent of agencies served a jurisdiction governed by a local board of health. In twenty-seven states, agencies operated purely as decentralized units of local government. The majority of top agency executives hold a master's degree; 29 percent have a bachelor's degree, and 17 percent have a doctorate.[21]

Federal Public Health Agencies

The federal public health system is composed primarily of the U.S. Department of Health and Human Services (HHS) and its operating divisions. Those of principal interest to state and local public health agencies are the CDC, the Health Resources and Services Administration, the Food and Drug Administration, the Centers for Medicare and Medicaid Services, and the Agency for Healthcare Research and Quality (figure 10.2). The agency with the greatest investment in nearly all states is the U.S. Department of Agriculture, with its Women, Infants, and Children (WIC) nutrition program. With regard to preparedness, one of the most important agencies that public health agencies work with at both the state and local levels is the Department of Homeland Security and, more specifically, the Federal Emergency Management Agency (FEMA). There are a number of other HHS operating divisions and other federal agencies in addition to those mentioned here that some state and local agencies work with, but with much less frequency.

HHS is the U.S. government's principal agency for protecting the health of all Americans and providing essential human services, especially for those who are least able to help themselves. HHS represents almost a quarter of all federal outlays, and it administers more grant dollars than all other federal agencies combined. The Medicare program is the nation's largest health insurer, handling more than 1 billion claims per year. Medicare and Medicaid together provide health care insurance for one in four Americans. HHS works closely with state and local governments, and many HHS-funded services are provided at the local level by state or county agencies or through private-sector grantees. The department's programs are administered by eleven operating divisions, including eight agencies in the U.S. Public Health Service and three human services agencies. The department includes more than 300 programs covering a wide spectrum of activities. In addition to the services they deliver, HHS programs ensure equitable treatment of beneficiaries nationwide, and they enable the collection of national health and other data. Departmental leadership is provided by the Office of the Secretary. The Program Support Center, a self-supporting division of the department, provides administrative services for HHS and other federal agencies.[22]

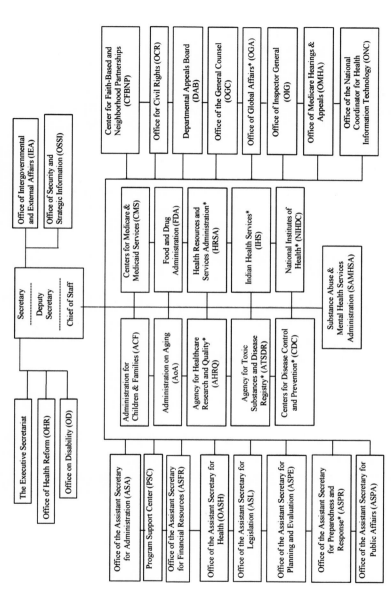

Figure 10.2. Hierarchy of agencies within the U.S. Department of Health and Human Services, July 2011. *Source:* www.hhs.gov/about/orgchart/.

*Designates a component of the U.S. Public Health Service

The boxes in the chart read:

The Executive Secretariat

Office of Health Reform (OHR)

Office on Disability (OD)

Office of Intergovernmental and External Affairs (IEA)

Office of Security and Strategic Information (OSSI)

Secretary

Deputy Secretary

Chief of Staff

Center for Faith-Based and Neighborhood Partnerships (CFBNP)

Office for Civil Rights (OCR)

Departmental Appeals Board (DAB)

Office of the General Counsel (OGC)

Office of Global Affairs* (OGA)

Office of Inspector General (OIG)

Office of Medicare Hearings & Appeals (OMHA)

Office of the National Coordinator for Health Information Technology (ONC)

Centers for Medicare & Medicaid Services (CMS)

Food and Drug Administration (FDA)

Health Resources and Services Administration* (HRSA)

Indian Health Services* (IHS)

National Institutes of Health* (NIHDC)

Substance Abuse & Mental Health Services Administration (SAMHSA)

Administration for Children & Families (ACF)

Administration on Aging (AoA)

Agency for Healthcare Research and Quality* (AHRQ)

Agency for Toxic Substances and Disease Registry* (ATSDR)

Centers for Disease Control and Prevention* (CDC)

Office of the Assistant Secretary for Administration (ASA)

Program Support Center (PSC)

Office of the Assistant Secretary for Financial Resources (ASFR)

Office of the Assistant Secretary for Health (OASH)

Office of the Assistant Secretary for Legislation (ASL)

Office of the Assistant Secretary for Planning and Evaluation (ASPE)

Office of the Assistant Secretary for Preparedness and Response* (ASPR)

Office of the Assistant Secretary for Public Affairs (ASPA)

Contemporary Efforts to Strengthen Public Health Organizations and Systems

A variety of initiatives are now under way to improve the effectiveness and efficiency of public health organizations and to achieve greater synergy and collective impact among the many organizations working within the public health system. Some of the most promising efforts are outlined here.

Performance standards

The National Public Health Performance Standards Program was developed at the CDC with national partners that included the ASTHO, NACCHO, National Association of Local Boards of Health (NALBOH), Public Health Foundation, and American Public Health Association (APHA). The goal of the program was to assess the capacity of state and local public health systems to provide the optimal level of public health. The program was based on the ten essential services of public health, and an expert consensus panel was used to develop standards, measures, and individual indicators that would be assessed using a community consensus model. This effort encouraged stakeholders to develop concrete plans to improve capacity and outline strategies for improving public health. Many saw it as the progenitor of public health agency accreditation.

Accreditation

With the support of the CDC and the Robert Wood Johnson Foundation and the leadership of organizational members ASTHO, NACCHO, NALBOH and APHA, the Public Health Accreditation Board (PHAB) was founded in 2007 (described more fully in chapter 7). Under this voluntary program, tribal, state, local, and territorial governmental public health agencies can choose to pursue accreditation. One of the most important considerations for the public is that a public health agency is in full compliance with the national standards established to ensure that it can carry out its functions. Agencies that seek accreditation are asked to conduct a rigorous self-study as well as submit to an on-site field review of their concurrence with the minimum standards for accreditation.

Quality improvement

Public health agencies, like all complex organizations, are faced with opportunities for improvement. Unlike many other components of the health sector, public health departments have not been early adopters of quality improvement initiatives. But with ever-increasing scrutiny of tighter budgets and more frequent demands for accountability, public health officials are now more interested in adopting strategies that improve organizational effectiveness and efficiency. To that end, the Robert Wood Johnson Foundation has sponsored several collaborative technical assistance activities for public health agencies to help them gain expertise and proficiency in quality improvement technology and methods. In addition, the CDC, NACCHO, and ASTHO provide support to health departments that want to incorporate quality improvement into their organizations. Proficiency and a demonstration of commitment to quality improvement are also requirements for organizations seeking national accreditation from PHAB.

Organizational reengineering

Closely related to quality improvement is the notion that, after a close examination of needs, resources, and current abilities, an organization may have to completely reconfigure its structure and operations in order to fulfill its mission. In this case, an organization may choose to undertake a fundamental redesign of staffing, work processes, and outputs rather than making incremental improvements to existing processes. Sometimes these changes are designed to improve efficiency, such as requiring fewer people to accomplish a particular task. Sometimes the process redesign requires new technology or a higher or different level of public health professional. All these adjustments—including changes to people, processes, and technology—come under the heading of organizational reengineering, or matching organizational resources with the needs of the mission.

These four developments in public health practice are occurring within a larger context of health system reform, creating additional opportunities for organizational change and improvement. The Patient Protection and Affordable Care Act of 2010 contained several provisions to reorganize medical care providers in ways that improve the quality and efficiency of care. For instance, accountable care organizations (ACOs) bring together multiple health care providers under a common organizational and financing framework to coordinate care and assume collective accountability for the health outcomes of defined populations of patients. Likewise, patient-centered medical home (PCMH) models are designed to integrate and coordinate the full range of services and supports needed by people to maintain health and well-being. The 2010 law also supports the expanded delivery of evidence-based preventive services and public health programs through a new dedicated, recurring federal fund. All these new provisions are being implemented alongside components of the health reform law that are designed to significantly expand health insurance coverage and reduce the number of American residents without coverage.

These elements of health reform create opportunities for public health organizations to negotiate new roles and responsibilities vis-à-vis their partners in medical care delivery. What roles should state and local health agencies play in the new ACO and PCMH models? Will these new structures, coupled with expanded health insurance coverage, allow public health agencies to move away from the direct delivery of clinical services? And if so, will agencies be able to reinvest the resources to strengthen other types of public health activities? How will these new organizational forms impact the multiorganizational relationships that currently exist within the public health system to support health assessment, planning, policy development, and program implementation? What new types of oversight and evaluation will emerge for public health agencies within the reforming health system? Public health agencies and their partners must forge the answers to these questions in the midst of challenging economic conditions, constrained budgets, and considerable political uncertainty. In doing so, public health agencies and their partners will be reinventing the public health system for the next generation of Americans.

Notes

1. Halverson PK, Miller CA, Kaluzny AD, Fried BJ, Schenck SE, Richards TB. Performing public health functions: The perceived contribution of public health and other community agencies. *J Health Human Services Administration.* 1996;18:288–303.

2. Mays GP, Halverson PK, Stevens R. The contributions of managed care plans to public health practice: Evidence from the nation's largest local health departments. *Public Health Rep.* 2001;116:50–67.

3. Mays GP, Miller CE, Halverson PK. *Local Public Health Practice: Trends and Models.* Washington, DC: American Public Health Association; 2000.

4. Halverson PK. Embracing the strength of the public health system: Why strong government public health agencies are vitally necessary but insufficient. *J Public Health Manag Pract.* 2002;8:98–100.

5. Mays GP, Halverson PK, Kaluzny AD. Collaboration to improve community health: Trends and alternative models. *Jt Comm J Qual Improv.* 1998;24:518–540.

6. Mays GP, Halverson PK, Baker EL, Stevens R, Vann JJ. Availability and perceived effectiveness of public health activities in the nation's most populous communities. *Am J Public Health.* 2004;94:1019–1026.

7. Institute of Medicine. *The Future of the Public's Health in the 21st Century.* Washington, DC: National Academies Press; 2002.

8. Beitsch LM, Brooks RG, Menachemi N, Libbey PM. Public health at center stage: New roles, old props. *Health Aff.* 2006;25:911–922.

9. Institute of Medicine. Committee for the Study of the Future of Public Health. *The Future of Public Health.* Washington, DC: National Academies Press; 1988.

10. Centers for Disease Control and Prevention. *National Public Health Standards Program User Guide.* Washington, DC: CDC; 2007.

11. Association of State and Territorial Health Officials. *Profile of State Public Health.* Vol. 2. Washington, DC: ASTHO; 2011.

12. Association of State and Territorial Health Officials. *Chartbook of Public Health.* Washington, DC: ASTHO; 2007.

13. Mays GP, Smith SA, Ingram RC, Racster LJ, Lamberth CD, Lovely ES. Public health delivery systems: Evidence, uncertainty, and emerging research needs. *Am J Prev Med.* 2009;36:256–265.

14. Honore PA, Amy BW. Public health finance: Fundamental theories, concepts, and definitions. *J Public Health Manag Pract.* 2007;13:89–92.

15. Mays GP, McHugh MC, Shim K, et al. Getting what you pay for: Public health spending and the performance of essential public health services. *J Public Health Manag Pract.* 2004;10:435–443.

16. Mays GP, McHugh MC, Shim K, et al. Institutional and economic determinants of public health system performance. *Am J Public Health.* 2006;96:523–531.

17. Mays GP, Smith SA. Geographic variation in public health spending: Correlates and consequences. *Health Serv Res.* 2009;44:1796–1817.

18. Mays GP, Smith SA. Evidence links increases in public health spending to declines in preventable deaths. *Health Aff.* 2011;30:1585–1593.

19. Association of State and Territorial Health Officials. *Budget Cuts Continue to Affect the Health of Americans: Update May 2011.* Washington, DC: ASTHO; 2011.

20. National Association of County and City Health Officials. *2005 National Profile of Local Health Departments.* Washington, DC: NACCHO; 2006.

21. National Association of County and City Health Officials. *2010 National Profile of Local Health Departments.* Washington, DC: NACCHO; 2011.

22. U.S. Department of Health and Human Services. About HHS. http://www.hhs.gov/about/. Accessed October 11, 2011.

11

International Lessons for the United States on Health, Health Care, and Health Policy

Stephen C. Schoenbaum, Robin Osborn, and David Squires

For many years, health care has been significantly more costly in the United States than in other countries. Nonetheless, overall U.S. health system performance and population outcomes often fall short of achievements in other countries.[1-3] Among sixteen member countries of the Organization for Economic Cooperation and Development (OECD), the United States had the highest death rate from conditions that are potentially preventable or treatable—the so-called mortality amenable to health care. Although the death rate from these conditions has decreased in each of these countries, the rate of decline was lower in the United States than elsewhere (figure 11.1).[4]

But within the United States there is also an enormous amount of variation in performance. Indeed, for an outcome such as "mortality amenable to health care, there are states within the U.S. (e.g., Minnesota) whose outcomes are as good as, if not better than, the best of the OECD countries."[5] And it is well known that one can receive excellent care at a variety of U.S. health care institutions. It is important to keep in mind that no single country or health care delivery system excels in every aspect of health care, health system performance, and health outcome. Ultimately, the objective is for the United States as a whole (and for other countries) to achieve increasingly better results and obtain greater value for its health care expenditures. To do so, it is important to examine best practices, wherever they occur.

In every country, multiple factors contribute to health outcomes, including (1) the prevalence and severity of illnesses in the population (particularly chronic conditions); (2) access to care and services when needed, including

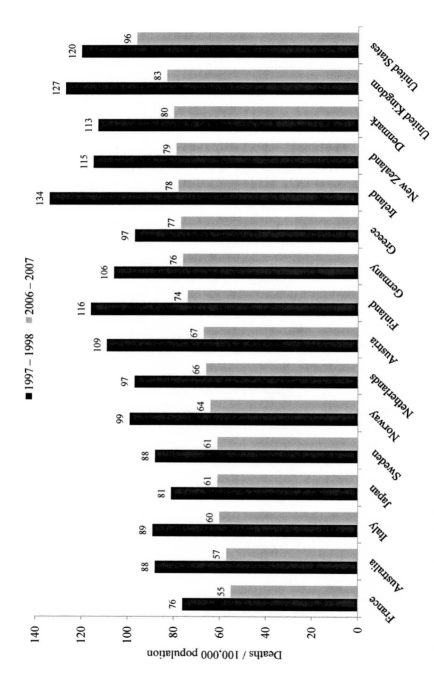

Figure 11.1. United States lags other countries in mortality amenable to health care. *Source:* Adapted from Nolte E, McKee M. Variations in amenable mortality—trends in 16 high-income nations. *Health Policy.* 2011;103(1):47–52.

preventive care, acute and transitional care, and chronic care; and (3) the effectiveness, safety, and efficiency of services when they are provided.

The prevalence and severity of chronic conditions are increasing in developed countries around the world, and the U.S. rates of chronic conditions and multiple chronic conditions are very high. In the 2005 Medical Expenditure Panel Survey, 55 percent of Americans aged 20 to 64 reported having no chronic conditions. In contrast, only one in eight Americans aged 65 and older (12.5 percent) reported having no chronic conditions, and disturbingly, almost half reported having three or more chronic conditions. In a similar survey, the percentage of Australians aged 65 and older who reported having no chronic conditions was also relatively low (18.4 percent), but the percentage of older Australians who reported having three or more chronic conditions was less than half the U.S. percentage (22.9 versus 47.6 percent).[6] Such results have significant implications not only for population outcomes but also for overall health care costs, public health programs, and health care delivery systems.

Among developed countries, the issue of large numbers of uninsured and underinsured has been unique to the United States. But with the advent of health care reform, the United States is on the threshold of implementing changes that will significantly reduce these numbers, which should have significant implications for health system performance.[7] For example, in 2005 about half the general population of adults in the United States reported receiving all recommended screening and preventive care for their age group, compared with only one-third of uninsured adults.[8] Among sick adults, one in two reported forgoing needed medical care because of the cost; that is, they did not see a doctor, did not fill a prescription, or failed to get recommended tests or follow-up care.[9] These gaps should be reduced by covering the uninsured and improving coverage for the underinsured. Indeed, there is direct evidence from the Oregon Health Insurance Experiment (a randomized study) that previously uninsured persons who gained coverage obtained more services than those who remained uninsured; the newly insured also reported better physical and mental health.[10]

The effectiveness of delivered health care services varies among countries and for different conditions within a country. For example, five-year survival rates for cancers vary both among and within countries. The United States has better five-year survival rates for breast and colorectal cancer compared with several other developed countries.[3] However, the five-year survival rate for cervical cancer is better in Canada (71.9 percent) and the Netherlands (69.0 percent) than in the United States (67.0 percent). These results are not simply a function of screening rates: the breast cancer screening rate is lower in the United States than in several other countries, whereas, the cervical cancer screening rate is higher in the United States than in Canada and the Netherlands.[2]

Best Practices

Broadly speaking, best practices related to health care and health system performance and improvement can be grouped in several categories: those having a strong primary care infrastructure and strong primary care services; those emphasizing prevention and population health; those providing comprehensive coverage and a value-based insurance design; those encouraging professional engagement in quality and providing aligned incentives for provider payment; and those consisting of a coherent national health care policy.

Primary care

Strong primary care services are associated with better outcomes, lower costs, and greater equity of care.[11] There are four characteristics of primary care services that contribute to these results: first contact care, continuity, comprehensiveness, and coordination. Excellent primary care leads to enhanced prevention services, including the early detection of illness; facilitated access to acute care; better chronic care, including patient education and engagement, monitoring, and effective and efficient use of health care and community services; and better transitional care, including referrals, medication reconciliation, and follow-up when patients change health care settings (e.g., when discharged from hospital to home).

In several countries, almost 100 percent of the population has a regular doctor or regular place of care, whereas this is true of only 91 percent in the United States.[12] Coverage for health care services is one factor contributing to this difference: persons with continuous health insurance coverage over the course of a year are more likely to report having a regular doctor or a regular place of care than are the uninsured—96 percent versus 77 percent (unpublished calculations by the authors). Other factors that might contribute to the lack of a regular health care provider include a frequent change in insurers, owing to patients changing jobs or employers changing benefits plans, or frequent relocation by both patients and physicians. In addition to having a regular doctor or place of care, more than 76 percent of chronically ill patients in the Netherlands, France, and Germany, had long-term relationships (five years or longer) with their primary care doctors. In contrast, only 53 percent of U.S. patients reported having similar long-term relationships. Again, the same factors (changes in insurers, jobs, or locations) are likely to account for these differences. Because long-term relationships and continuity of care are associated with greater trust and better outcomes,[13, 14] it is important to address mutable factors that might lead to discontinuities in care.

In several countries (Australia, Denmark, England, the Netherlands), primary care physicians play a gatekeeper role, and in these countries, this is not seen as a negative. In the managed care era of the 1990s, however, the American public interpreted gatekeeping as being synonymous with rationing. This reaction may have reflected the fact that Americans were accustomed to having free choice of providers and unlimited access to specialists and second opinions. This pattern has been reinforced by the disproportionately small percentage of primary care doctors versus specialists in the United States compared with other countries. This has the effect of channeling patients directly to specialty care without referrals. Another explanation of this different reaction to gatekeeping may be related to the fact that primary care physicians in other countries are seen as facilitators and coordinators of necessary care, rather than as barriers to desired care. In addition, primary care physicians in other countries are not perceived as deriving any direct financial benefit from withholding care—a major concern related to managed care in the United States. In countries where primary care gatekeeping has not been built into the system, such as France and Germany, "soft gatekeeping" models are being promoted: patients are encouraged to register with a primary care doctor or practice and may receive a financial incentive in the form of reduced cost-sharing. In Ontario, Canada, a wave of innovative practice models were implemented as part of an effort to reinforce primary care and more comprehensive care; as a result, more than 70 percent of the population has voluntarily enrolled with a primary care provider.[15]

With respect to well-developed primary care services, Denmark provides some interesting examples. A 1998 Eurobarometer survey showed that 90 percent of Danes were satisfied with their health care services, a greater proportion than in any other member of the European Union.[16] Ninety-nine percent of Danes choose a general practitioner (GP) as their gatekeeper. Only 1 percent has chosen to retain the system, prevalent until the 1970s, in which they have no gatekeeper and can see specialists without referral. This 1 percent must pay their physicians the difference between what the physician charges and what the government generally pays the physician for a visit.

GPs in Denmark have regular weekday office hours. The day generally starts with a telephone hour from 8:00 to 9:00 AM and concludes by about 3:00 PM. GPs are paid partially by capitation for persons enrolled in their practices and partially on a fee-for-service (FFS) basis, including fees for face-to-face visits, telephone encounters, and e-mail encounters (they receive more for e-mail encounters than for telephone encounters). Denmark also has a nationally mandated, regionally organized, physician-run service that operates when the GPs' offices are normally closed. This out-of-hours service is staffed by GPs, and they receive additional payment for participating. Danish GPs seem highly satisfied with their practice. Because there is a national health information exchange, they receive information from their patients' out-of-hours service encounters by the next business morning, and patients know that they can contact their GPs to provide or coordinate appropriate follow-up care. Similarly, when a patient is registered in the emergency department, Danish primary care physicians are automatically notified electronically.

When a GP refers a patient to a specialist, the patient can make an appointment with the specialist of his or her choice and can schedule the appointment through the national health information exchange. When the encounter occurs, the specialist enters information about the consultation in a specified format in order to receive payment. This information is available to the GP, who can then coordinate appropriate follow-up care.[17]

Several of the features of primary care in Denmark can be observed in other countries, and some are becoming more common in the United States. For example, the use of electronic medical records is nearly universal in many countries, including New Zealand, Australia, the Netherlands, and the United Kingdom (figure 11.2).[18] Electronic capabilities that are widely available in these countries include making lists of patients by diagnosis or laboratory result, receiving decision support to provide guideline-based interventions or screening tests, and sending patients reminders for preventive or follow-up care. One example of the use of advanced health information technology to improve the quality of patient care comes from New Zealand. GPs there use cardiovascular disease and diabetes assessment and management systems in which data fields are automatically prepopulated from the patient's electronic health record (EHR). The patient's risks are assessed through a decision-support tool, and treatment options are saved back into the EHR. GPs then receive risk-assessed, patient-specific, evidence-based advice at the time of care.[19, 20]

The United States lags behind on electronic health information capabilities, with fewer than half of primary care physicians reporting the use of electronic medical records in 2009 and even fewer reporting additional capabilities (table 11.1). Nonetheless, thanks to the American Recovery and Reinvestment Act of 2009 (the "stimulus bill") the adoption and use of electronic medical records have accelerated greatly.[21, 22] As a result of a combination of positive and negative incentives that are being built into Medicare system, within a few years, most drug prescribing in the United States should be electronic. This has

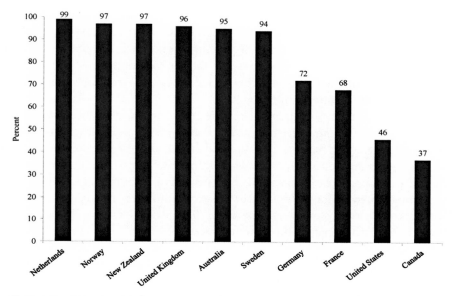

Figure 11.2. Percentage of primary care doctors using electronic patient medical records, 2009. *Source:* 2009 Commonwealth Fund International Health Policy Survey of Primary Care Physicians.

Table 11.1. Primary Care Doctors' Computerized Capacity to Generate Patient Information by Country, 2009

Percentage Reporting the Computerized Capacity to Generate:	Aus	Can	Fr	Ger	Neth	NZ	Swe	UK	US
List of patients by diagnosis	93	73	20	82	73	97	74	90	42
List of patients by lab result	88	23	15	56	62	84	67	85	29
List of patients who are due or overdue to tests or preventive care	95	22	19	65	69	96	41	89	29
List of all medications taken by an individual patient	94	25	24	65	61	96	49	86	30

Source: 2009 Commonwealth Fund International Health Policy Survey of Primary Care Physicians.

been the case in Denmark for several years; prescriptions are not only trans-
ferred directly to the pharmacy of the patient's choice but also linked to mechanisms that can virtually eliminate dispensing errors (such as matching the bar
code generated by the physician's order to the bar code of the medication dis-
pensed). Bar-code matching is becoming more common in the United States,
but it still occurs primarily in hospitals.

In many countries, multidisciplinary primary care teams are the norm, with
nurses and other nonphysician health care professionals typically sharing responsibility for managing patients' care. In Sweden, the United Kingdom, the Netherlands, Australia, and New Zealand, such team-based care is nearly universal in
primary care practices, compared with 59 percent of U.S. primary care doctors
reporting shared responsibility. One of Ontario's innovative primary care models
consists of the establishment of more than 170 family health teams. These teams
include family physicians, who continue to see their own patients during regular
office hours, plus "other health care professionals . . . such as nurse practitioners,
nurses, dieticians and pharmacists" and "access to a Family Health Team doctor during extended evening and weekend hours for urgent problems."[23] When a
patient is seen by another physician or after hours, his or her own physician receives a written summary by the next day (with the patient's permission).

Because traditional payment methods such as FFS are often accused of
hindering the coordination of care, financial incentives can be offered to encourage and reward primary care physicians for managing patients with
chronic diseases or complex health care needs, who often see many different
physicians and follow multiple medication regimens. More than half of physicians report being eligible for these incentives in several countries, including
82 percent of physicians in the United Kingdom, compared with only 17 percent in the United States (table 11.2).[18]

Finding after-hours care is a problem in several countries, where between
one-third and two-thirds of patients reported difficulty getting care on nights,
weekends, or holidays without going to an emergency room (figure 11.3).[24]
The best results were in the Netherlands, where only 33 percent of adults surveyed reported that it was "very or somewhat difficult" to get non–emergency
room care after hours, versus 63 percent in the United States and France, 65
percent in Canada, and 68 percent in Sweden. The Netherlands, like Denmark, now has a mandatory, regionally organized off-hours service.[25] As an
alternative to providing coverage through a self-organized rotation of doctors,
since the early 2000s, GP-led cooperatives have been set up around the Netherlands, covering more than 90 percent of the population. Increasingly colo-
cated at hospitals, they provide telephone triage by trained nurses and medical
assistants using national guidelines and protocols, GP backup for telephone

Table 11.2. Financial Incentives and Targeted Support in Primary Care, by Country, 2009

Percentage Eligible to Receive Financial Incentives for:	Aus	Can	Fr	Ger	Neth	NZ	Swe	UK	US
High patient satisfaction ratings	29	1	2	4	4	2	4	49	19
Achieving clinical care targets	25	21	6	6	23	74	5	84	28
Managing patients with chronic diseases or complex needs	53	54	42	48	61	55	2	82	17
Enhancing preventive care activities	28	26	14	23	17	38	2	37	10
Adding nonphysician clinicians to practice	38	21	3	17	60	19	2	26	6
Non–face-to-face interactions with patients	10	16	3	7	35	5	4	17	7

Source: 2009 Commonwealth Fund International Health Policy Survey of Primary Care Physicians.

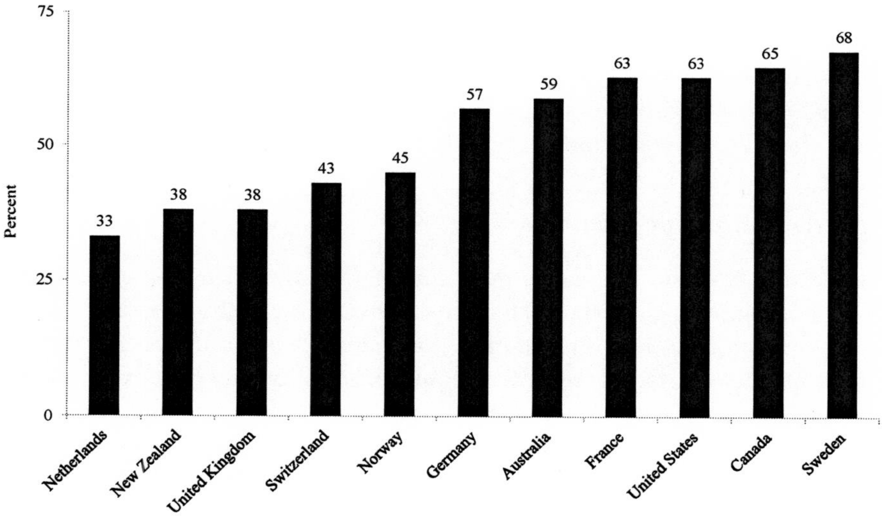

Figure 11.3. Percentage of respondents who found it very/somewhat difficult to get after-hours care (nights, weekends, holidays) without going to the emergency room, 2010. *Source:* 2010 Commonwealth Fund International Health Policy Survey in Eleven Countries.

consultations and walk-in visits, and GP home visits with medically equipped vehicles. EHRs are created and sent to the patient's regular GP. GP satisfaction is high, as their average hours on call dropped from nineteen to four per week. One study in the Netherlands showed that such a service reduces the use of emergency rooms for problems that can be handled in other settings.[26]

The good news in the United States is that there is now a movement to promote the development of medical homes. The National Committee for Quality Improvement (NCQA) recognizes primary care practices that meet the criteria for being medical homes.[27] In addition, the Affordable Care Act of 2010 and a variety of private efforts are stimulating the development of accountable care organizations (ACOs). ACOs are required to have a strong primary care base, and since they are accountable for the quality and cost of care, there is a great incentive for them to provide services to primary care practices that enable them to serve as medical homes and gain access to specialty and ancillary care in a manner that is effective, efficient, and coordinated.[28]

Programs such as Community Care of North Carolina (CCNC) have decreased the use of emergency services and reduced hospitalizations. CCNC provides fourteen regional networks of physicians with incentive payments to hire care managers to provide coordinated and preventive care for Medicaid patients with chronic illnesses. An analysis by an outside consultant found that CCNC saved nearly $1.5 billion in health care costs from 2007 through 2009.[29] Similarly, Bridges to Excellence is a multistate, multiple-employer initiative that has demonstrated cost savings; it gives primary care physicians incentives for providing medical homes and adhering to medical guidelines to monitor and treat chronic conditions such as diabetes and hypertension.[30]

Prevention and population health

Interestingly, health outcomes in Denmark (as assessed by life expectancy and other indices of mortality) have not been as good as those in several other European countries.[4] In the past, the Danish population has had higher rates of smoking, fat intake, and alcohol consumption and lower rates of exercise,[31] despite Denmark's excellent primary care infrastructure. These results were apparently attributable to the lack of well-developed national goals and programs targeted at prevention and population health. Denmark has acknowledged the problem and is developing new national programs targeted at smoking and other significant health issues, as well as participating in an OECD health care quality indicators project that emphasizes prevention practices in primary care.[32]

Recognizing the importance of prevention, several countries reward primary care physicians for offering "enhanced" preventive care services, such as patient counseling and group visits; 38 percent of physicians reported being able to receive such incentives in New Zealand, and 37 percent in the United Kingdom (see table 11.2).[18] Following a 2002 reform, physician-based and patient-centered disease management programs were implemented nationwide in Germany. Over the years, programs have been developed and implemented for type 1 and type 2 diabetes, breast cancer, asthma and chronic obstructive pulmonary disease (COPD), and coronary heart disease. Integral features of these programs include information technology support; a central role for the patient's primary care physician; a patient-centered approach that supports patient self-management; quality assurance, including reminders and benchmarking; and financial incentives for doctors, patients, and sickness funds (private health insurers). The German government provides payments to each of the sickness funds, based on the number of people enrolled in the disease management programs. In turn, the sickness funds provide financial incentives to primary care physicians to enroll eligible patients. All the insurers use the same government-specified, evidence-based guidelines. Despite what is otherwise a comparatively weak primary care system, early results for diabetic patients showed that quality of care and patient satisfaction improved, while mortality, hospitalization rates, complications, and both drug and hospital costs went down compared with other insured patients.[33]

The United States does comparatively well when it comes to prevention, although, as previously noted, there is room for significant improvement. National guidelines have been established by bodies such as the U.S. Preventive Services Task Force and the Centers for Disease Control and Prevention's Advisory Committee on Immunization Practices. Nongovernmental committees and organizations have also developed guidelines, such as the American Academy of Pediatrics' Redbook Committee, the American Cancer Society, and the American Heart Association. These various guidelines may not always be in agreement, but there is greater standardization in prevention than in several other areas of clinical and public health practice. The availability of guidelines has made it possible to develop measures of performance and implement them widely. For example, for more than fifteen years, the Healthcare Effectiveness Data and Information Set of the NCQA has been used to assess health plan performance on a variety of screening, prevention, and chronic disease management practices. Each year the NCQA issues a report on the state of health care quality, and performance on most of the measures has improved significantly.[34]

Table 11.3. Cost-Related Access Problems among Chronically Ill Adults in the Past Two Years, by Country, 2008

Percentage of Patients Who:	Aus	Can	Fr	Ger	Neth	NZ	UK	US
Did not fill a prescription or skipped doses	20	18	13	12	3	18	7	43
Did not visit a doctor despite having a medical problem	21	9	11	15	3	22	4	36
Did not get a recommended test, treatment, or follow-up	25	11	13	13	3	18	6	38
Had any of the above access problems because of cost	36	25	23	26	7	31	13	54

Source: 2008 Commonwealth Fund International Health Policy Survey of Sicker Adults.

Comprehensive coverage and value-based insurance

Although coverage of the entire population is a necessary condition for a high-performing health system, it is not sufficient. Besides universality, there are several other facets that can contribute to higher performance. Effectiveness can be enhanced by minimizing cost sharing for the sickest and neediest members of a population so that they are more likely to get the care and treatments, such as medications, they need (table 11.3). In addition, efficiency can be enhanced by policies such as tiered co-pays for medications, based on their cost-effectiveness.

Because of the sheer complexity of insurance plans and the multitude of insurers, patients and doctors in the United States spend far more time dealing with insurance than do their counterparts in other countries. Half of U.S. primary care doctors reported that the time spent dealing with insurance restrictions on treatments was a major problem, compared with merely 6 percent in the United Kingdom. A 2011 study found that primary care physicians in the United States spent $82,975 a year interacting with payers, compared with $22,205 for Ontario physicians.[35] Similarly, nearly one-fifth of U.S. adults reported spending a significant amount of time on insurance paperwork or disputes over bills in the past year, and one-fourth reported that their insurance had denied payment or paid less than expected. Only 4 to 6 percent of respondents reported either of these problems in Sweden, the United Kingdom, and New Zealand.

Other countries use value-based benefits design in a wide variety of ways to remove financial barriers to access to "high-value services"—those for which the benefits outweigh the costs—and to discourage people from using "low-value services"—those for which the costs outweigh the benefits.[36] For example, in France, patients with any one of thirty chronic conditions are exempt from co-pays for primary care visits. In Germany, patients who enroll in disease management programs are exempt from cost sharing. In France, Sweden, Germany, and the Netherlands, children's primary care visits are exempt from co-pays. For prescription drugs, France has no co-pays for highly effective drugs and tiered co-pays for drugs with less therapeutic value.[36]

Some insurers and large employers in the United States are using value-based benefits design.[37, 38] For example, they are eliminating co-pays for certain drugs, such as those that treat hypertension or depression, and imposing higher co-pays for procedures considered to be of low value.

Professionalism and support for effective and efficient practices

There is increasing recognition that maintaining the highest standard of professionalism among physicians and other health care providers is extremely important for the performance of a health system. In 2002 leading U.S. and U.K. medical journals simultaneously published a document entitled "Medical Professionalism in the New Millennium: A Physician Charter," which was authored by the American Board of Internal Medicine, the American College of Physicians Foundation, and the European Federation of Internal Medicine.[39, 40] The charter has now been endorsed by more than 100 medical organizations around the world. "Its fundamental principles [are] the primacy of patient welfare, patient autonomy and social justice. The Charter articulates professional commitments of physicians and health care professionals, including improving access to high quality health care, advocating for a just and cost-effective distribution of finite resources, and maintaining trust by managing conflicts of interest."[41] Physicians and other health practitioners can enhance their professional behavior by taking advantage of several types of support to help them deliver more effective and efficient care. These include the development and deployment of clinical guidelines, feedback on patient clinical outcomes, clinical audits, and regular reviews of performance, including peer reviews.

Several countries embed treatment guidelines into primary care practice through financial incentives, electronic reminders and decision support, and professionally led efforts to translate evidence into practice. In the United Kingdom, the National Institute for Health and Clinical Excellence supports GP practices with more than seventy clinical guidelines covering primary prevention, diagnosis and treatment, and long-term follow-up for major diseases such as diabetes, hypertension, and schizophrenia.[42] More than 90 percent of U.K. doctors routinely use guidelines for diabetes, asthma or COPD, and

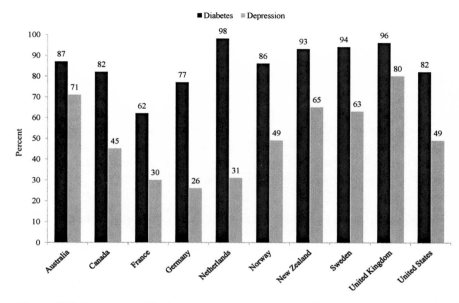

Figure 11.4. Percentage of primary care practices routinely using written treatment guidelines, by condition, 2009. *Source:* 2009 Commonwealth Fund International Health Policy Survey of Primary Care Physicians.

hypertension. A high percentage of doctors in New Zealand also use clinical guidelines. That country's Best Practice Advocacy Center—a physician-led nongovernmental, nonprofit organization—develops evidence-based clinical guidelines along with case studies, laboratory and prescribing reports, and a clinical audit package; it reaches out to primary care practices nationwide with campaigns, tools, and support to encourage adoption of its clinical guidelines.[43] Other leading countries in the use of clinical guidelines are Australia and the Netherlands. Notably, the use of treatment guidelines for conditions such as diabetes and asthma is more common than for depression, although large majorities of primary care physicians in the United Kingdom, Australia, New Zealand, and Sweden reported using such guidelines for depression as well (figure 11.4).[18]

Large majorities of Dutch, Swedish, and New Zealand physicians receive feedback on outcomes, reflecting national strategies to focus on examples of high performance and on areas for improvement. The United Kingdom is a leader in using performance measurement and feedback in relation to benchmarks for quality improvement in primary care: 96 percent of primary care physicians reported receiving and reviewing data on patient experience, and

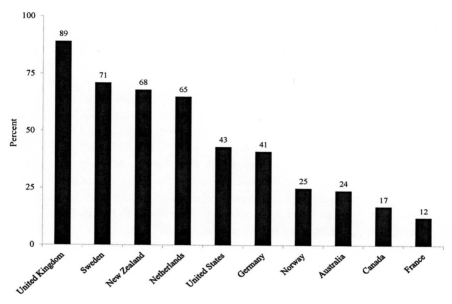

Figure 11.5. Percentage of primary care practices routinely receiving and reviewing data on patient clinical outcomes, 2009. *Source:* 2009 Commonwealth Fund International Health Policy Survey of Primary Care Physicians.

89 percent reviewed data on patient outcomes (figure 11.5); 92 percent reported that their clinical performance is reviewed annually against targets; and 65 percent received data comparing their performance with that of other practitioners. A major driver for these results has been the GP contract, which is described in the next section on financial incentives.

In addition, for more than a decade the United Kingdom has been working to introduce a process called revalidation, which is equivalent to the relicensure of physicians.[44,45] The objective is to link revalidation to ongoing assessments of physician performance and to programs to improve performance that are tailored to individual physician needs. Instruments for regular review of physician performance have been developed and are being tested, and implementation is expected to begin in late 2012 for all practicing physicians.[46]

Financial incentives

Several countries are using their payment systems to encourage and support better clinical performance. In England and the Netherlands, where capitation is the predominant method of physician payment, new blended models that include FFS and pay-for-performance (P4P) incentives have been introduced. In Australia and Canada, where FFS is the predominant method of payment, elements of capitation or incentive payments have been incorporated to achieve better results. Similarly, the United States seems to be headed toward blended payment models. By far, the most common method of payment for physician services is FFS. Hospitals are paid by diagnosis-related group (DRG), which entails a single bundled payment for acute hospital services for a particular diagnosis code; per diem, which is a flat daily rate that depends on whether the patient is receiving intensive care or regular care; or FFS. Attempts to capitate payments to physicians in the managed care era of the 1990s failed in most instances. Physicians were often asked to take on more financial risk than was prudent for them to assume. Recently, as the United States has entered the era of health care reform and ACOs, it is likely that capitation will be reintroduced, along with methods for mitigating the financial risks, such as risk-adjusted payments and reinsurance. In addition, payers are introducing bundled payments that are more complex than DRGs—for example, payments that provide a lump sum not just for hospital services for a particular condition but also for associated physician and other services before and after hospitalization.[47] Bundling payments and ultimately paying for care by capitation will give providers an incentive to deliver care efficiently.

One type of P4P that is related to efficiency is based on shared savings between insurers and providers. When a predetermined amount is expected to be spent on providers' services but the actual amount paid by the insurer is less, in accordance with a prior agreement, the savings are divided and shared.[48] Nonetheless, P4P is used predominantly to give providers an incentive to deliver more effective care—that is, to meet various performance measures that are often related to quality of care (see table 11.2).[47] Primary care doctors in Australia are encouraged to improve the quality of care through financial incentives. Faced with serious challenges in fragmented primary health care in the FFS environment, the Australian Department of Health and Ageing introduced practice incentives payments (PIPs) in 1998 as part of a broader strategy of reform. These PIPs reward physicians in thirteen areas, including comprehensive after-hours care, rural practices, teaching of medical students, and use of EHRs. Practices choose which of the incentive areas to participate in. Incentive payments averaged $61,600 per practice in 2008–2009.[49]

The United Kingdom has also been a leader in using P4P to drive quality improvement. In 2004, P4P was introduced as part of a general medical services contract designed to reward practices for the provision of quality care and to standardize improvements in the delivery of clinical care. Considered the largest P4P experiment in the world, the program includes 136 quality indicators covering four domains (clinical, organizational, patient experiences, additional services). Payments are based on the proportion of patients achieving the quality target, and GPs can receive amounts up to 25 percent of their income. Most of the payments are linked to evidence-based process measures for the management of chronic disease.[50]

Coherent National Policies

Ferlie and Shortell have promulgated the principle that to improve health care and health throughout a country, simultaneous efforts at multiple levels are required, including the individual, group or team, organization, and larger environment or system.[51] They urge that "attention be given to issues of leadership, culture, team development, and information technology at all levels."[51] To address the larger environment or system, national policies are both useful and essential. Ideally, these policies form a coherent whole, albeit one that is tractable to periodic assessment and improvement. Although this chapter has already examined several national policies, a closer look at the Netherlands and England is in order.

In the Netherlands, sharply rising health care costs highlighted the need for a coherent national policy and vision for the health sector. A number of reforms were initiated beginning in 1974 to increase the government's influence on health care, to move toward a single national health insurance scheme for all citizens (at the time, coverage was split between compulsory social insurance through sickness funds for lower-income workers and voluntary private health insurance for higher-income citizens), and to strengthen primary care. Although there were incremental changes, not all the reforms succeeded. Debate continued until 2006, when a sweeping structural reform was implemented. This involved compulsory private insurance coverage for all citizens, a regulated form of managed competition among the country's private insurers, and a change in the role of government from direct control of volume, prices, and capacity to "setting the rules of the game."[52] Although the Dutch Ministry of Health, Welfare, and Sport defines the policies that guarantee access to high-quality health care facilities and services and is responsible for ensuring the health sector's performance, the insurers and providers of care are private. To carry out a coherent national vision for health care, the government delegates certain roles and tasks to key quasi-governmental supervisory and advisory authorities, including the Dutch Health Care Insurance Board, an independent agency that advises the ministry on the basic health insurance package and administers the risk-adjustment program, comparative effectiveness, and long-term care insurance; the Dutch Health Care Authority, an independent administrative body funded by the ministry with responsibility for supervising health care markets and setting prices and budgets for most health care providers; the Dutch Health Inspectorate, also independent from the ministry, which supervises the quality and accessibility of health care; and the Dutch Competition Authority, which operates across all sectors of the economy to prevent cartels, assess market consolidation, and avert abuse by a dominant market position.[53, 54] Operating within broad legislative frameworks, these authorities are key to operationalizing a coherent national policy. They are designed to enable flexible, timely, and politically sheltered decision making and, at the same time, ensure accountability, stakeholder input, and transparency. Through these relatively independent, quasi-governmental authorities that together address access, quality, and costs, the Dutch government is able to achieve its public goals and implement the principles of national health care reform.[52]

In England, the vision for health reform and its implementation can be similarly traced. It consists of setting out a broad national policy and establishing key institutions and entities to oversee the operationalization of that policy. Following the 1997 election, the Blair government undertook a system-wide reform, which was outlined in a series of white papers. These began in 2000 with the National Health Service (NHS) plan, which laid out a plan for the twenty-first century.[55] The scope of the reforms was sweeping, underpinned by an infusion of funding that would increase the NHS budget by 43 percent in real terms over the first five years and include major investments in workforce and facilities, national standards and national inspections, evidence-based practice, payment reform to reward quality and performance, consumer choice and guaranteed access to care, and innovative delivery models for primary care and chronic conditions. To take its pledge for reform forward, the government instituted an array of national initiatives, programs, and quasi-governmental authorities, including an ambitious P4P contract for GPs; the establishment of national performance targets and national service frameworks that set priorities for improvement and established standards of care for conditions, such as diabetes or cancer, or for vulnerable populations, such as the elderly; an initiative to give patients a choice of provider; and a program of public reporting of patient experiences and hospital performance indicators. Structural reforms included the creation of primary care trusts to promote more effective commissioning of care and greater accountability for resources devoted to the total care of patients; foundation trusts to give hospitals more operational independence, create greater accountability, and allow them to adapt services to local needs; and the introduction of NHS Direct, a national nurse-led telephone medical advice line to expand access to care. A number of quasi-independent agencies were also established to implement, oversee, and regulate quality and costs in the NHS, including the National Institute for Health and Clinical Excellence to conduct research on clinical effectiveness, produce and disseminate clinical practice guidelines, and inform coverage decisions and benefits design; Connecting for Health, a national health information technology strategy; the National Patient Safety Agency to identify and address patient safety issues; the Healthcare Commission (originally the Commission for Healthcare Audit and Inspection) to independently assess the performance of health system providers, investigate serious failures in health services, and publish ratings of NHS trusts; the NHS Institute for Innovation and Improvement to support evaluation, new ways of delivering patient-centered care, and the system-wide spread of successful innovations to re-engineer services; and Monitor, an independent regulator of foundation trusts to ensure quality of care and financial soundness. Not all these efforts were successful, and some will be dismantled in the next wave of reforms being implemented under Prime Minister Cameron. However, in combination, the reforms initiated by the Blair government revolutionized the NHS and pushed the system toward higher performance and significant improvements in access, quality, and accountability—all in a short time.[56, 57]

Concluding Comments

The health and health care of the U.S. population can be improved. Because of the wide variation in health system performance, it is possible to find a variety of best practices that merit widespread replication. Examples from other countries provide ample evidence of performance-improving practices that can be adapted and adopted without having to reinvent the wheel. One major difference between the United States and other developed countries is the lack of a coherent national health and health care policy and the lack of a ministry of health to oversee the health and health care of the country as a whole. Indeed, under our federal form of government, the states are responsible for many health and health care functions, and over the years, the development of a pluralistic, privately based set of organizations and agencies with responsibility for oversight of various parts of the health care system has made it difficult to establish coherent national policies. Nonetheless, the Affordable Care Act of 2010 could mark the beginning of a movement toward more national, or at least nationally coordinated, approaches to health and health care policy. The objectives of achieving better health and health care can and should be translated into measurable outcomes—a key first step in providing a clear focus for all public and private efforts.

Notes

1. Davis K, Schoen C, Stremikis K. *Mirror, Mirror on the Wall: How the Performance of the U.S. Health Care System Compares Internationally. 2010 Update.* Commonwealth Fund; June 2010. http://www.commonwealthfund.org/~/media/Files/Publications/Fund%20Report/2010/Jun/1400_Davis_Mirror_Mirror_on_the_wall_2010.pdf.

2. Anderson GF, Markovich P. *Multinational Comparisons of Health Systems Data, 2010.* Commonwealth Fund; July 2011. http://www.commonwealthfund.org/~/media/Files/Publications/Issue%20Brief/2011/Jul/PDF_1533_Anderson_multinational_comparisons_2010_OECD_pfd.pdf.

3. Squires DA. *The U.S. Health System in Perspective: A Comparison of Twelve Industrialized Nations.* Commonwealth Fund; July 2011. http://www.commonwealthfund.org/~/media/Files/Publications/Issue%20Brief/2011/Jul/1532_Squires_US_hlt_sys_comparison_12_nations_intl_brief_v2.pdf.

4. Nolte E, McKee M. Variations in amenable mortality—trends in 16 high-income nations. *Health Policy.* 2011;103(1):47–52.

5. Schoenbaum SC, Schoen C, Nicholson JL, Cantor JC. Mortality amenable to health care in the United States: The roles of demographics and health systems performance. *J Public Health Policy.* 2011;32(4):407–429.

6. Australian Institute of Health and Welfare. Health and welfare statistics and information—chronic diseases. http://www.aihw.gov.au/chronic-diseases.

7. U.S. Senate. The Patient Protection and Affordable Care Act: Detailed Summary. http://dpc.senate.gov/healthreformbill/healthbill04.pdf. Accessed September 10, 2011.

8. The Commonwealth Fund Commission on a High Performance Health System. *Why Not the Best? Results from the National Scorecard on U.S. Health System Performance, 2008.* Commonwealth Fund; July 2008. http://www.commonwealthfund.org/~/media/Files/Publications/Fund%20Report/2008/Jul/. Accessed September 26, 2011.

9. Schoen C, Osborn R, How SK, Doty MM, Peugh J. In chronic condition: Experiences of patients with complex health care needs, in eight countries, 2008. *Health Aff.* 2009;28(1):w1–w16.

10. Finkelstein A, Taubman S, Wright B, Bernstein M, Gruber J, Newhouse JP, Allen H, Baicker K, the Oregon Health Study Group. The Oregon Health Insurance Experiment: Evidence from the first year. NBER Working Paper No. 17190. July 2011. http://papers.nber.org/papers/w17190#fromrss. Accessed August 14, 2011.

11. Starfield B, Shi L, Macinko J. Contribution of primary care to health systems and health. *Milbank Q.* 2005;83(3):457–502.

12. Schoen C, Osborn R, Squires D, Doty MM, Pierson R, Applebaum S. Complex

health care needs in fragmented systems: Experiences in eleven countries, 2011. *Health Aff.* forthcoming. Note that the base includes only "sicker" patients with complex health care needs—see the article's technical appendix for details. The percentage with a regular doctor or regular place of care mirrors results from a 2007 survey of the general population.

13. Donahue KE, Ashkin E, Pathman DE. Length of patient-physician relationship and patients' satisfaction and preventive service use in the rural South: A cross-sectional telephone study. *BMC Fam Pract.* 2005;6:40. http://www.biomedcentral.com/1471-2296/6/40.

14. Hollander MJ, Kadlec H, Hamdi R, Tessaro A. Increasing value for money in the Canadian healthcare system: New findings on the contribution of primary care services. *Healthcare Q.* 2009;12(4):30–42.

15. Hutchison B, Levesque JF, Strumpf E, Coyle N. Primary health care in Canada: Systems in motion. *Milbank Q.* 2011;89(2):256–288.

16. Institute for the Study of Civil Society. Background briefing: Health care lessons from Denmark (2002). http://www.civitas.org.uk/pdf/Denmark.pdf. Accessed August 14, 2011.

17. Protti D, Johansen I. *Widespread Adoption of Information Technology in Primary Care Physician Offices in Denmark: A Case Study.* Commonwealth Fund; March 2010. http://www.commonwealthfund.org/~/media/Files/Publications/Issue%20Brief/2010/Mar/1379_Protti_widespread_adoption_IT_primary_care_Denmark_intl_ib.pdf.

18. Schoen C, Osborn R, Doty MM, Squires D, Peugh J, Applebaum S. A survey of primary care physicians in eleven countries, 2009: Perspectives on care, costs, and experiences. *Health Aff.* 2009;28(6):w1171–w1173.

19. Gray BH, Bowden T, Johansen I, Koch S. *Electronic Health Records: An International Perspective on "Meaningful Use."* Commonwealth Fund; November 2011. http://www.commonwealthfund.org/~/media/Files/Publications/Issue%20Brief/2011/Nov/1565_Gray_electronic_med_records_meaningful_use_intl_brief.pdf. Accessed May 21, 2012.

20. Protti D, Bowden T. *Electronic Medical Record Adoption in New Zealand Primary Care Physician Offices.* Commonwealth Fund; August 2010. http://www.commonwealthfund.org/~/media/Files/Publications/Issue%20Brief/2010/Aug/1434_Protti_electronic_med_record_adoption_New_Zealand_intl_brief.pdf.

21. The American Recovery and Reinvestment Act of 2009. http://frwebgate.access.gpo.gov/cgi-bin/getdoc.cgi?dbname=111_cong_bills&docid=f:h1enr.pdf. Accessed September 6, 2011.

22. Centers for Medicare and Medicaid Services. CMS EHR meaningful use overview. https://www.cms.gov/ehrincentiveprograms/30_Meaningful_Use.asp. Accessed September 6, 2011.

23. Ontario Ministry of Health and Long-Term Care. Understanding family health teams. http://www.health.gov.on.ca/transformation/fht/fht_understanding.html.

24. Schoen C, Osborn R, Squires D, Doty MM, Pierson R, Applebaum S. How health insurance design affects access to care and costs, by income, in eleven countries. *Health Aff.* 2010;29(12):2323–2334.

25. Huibers L, Giesen P, Wensing M, Grol R. Out-of-hours care in Western countries: Assessment of different organizational models. *BMC Health Serv Res.* 2009;9:105.

26. van Uden CJ, Winkens RA, Wesseling G, Fiolet HF, van Schayck OC, Crebolder HF. The impact of a primary care physician cooperative on the caseload of an emergency department: The Maastricht integrated out-of-hours service. *J Gen Intern Med.* 2005;20(7):612–617.

27. National Committee for Quality Assurance. Patient centered medical home. http://www.ncqa.org/tabid/631/default.aspx. Accessed September 26, 2011.

28. Schoenbaum SC. Accountable care organizations: Roles and opportunities for hospitals. *Hosp Pract (Minneapolis).* 2011;39(3):140–148.

29. Community Care of North Carolina. Our results. http://www.communitycarenc .org/our-results. Accessed September 30, 2011.

30. Center for Health Transformation. Bridges to Excellence. http://www .healthtransformation.net/cs/bridges_to_excellence. Accessed September 30, 2011.

31. Rosdahl N. Denmark: Concerned and yet content with itself. *Euro Observer.* 2001;3(1):7–8. http://www2.1se.ac.uk/LSEHealthAndSocialCare/LSEHealth/pdf/ euroObserver/Obsv013n01.pdf. Accessed August 14, 2011.

32. OECD health care quality indicators. http://www.oecd.org/document/34/0,37 46,en_2649_37407_37088930_1_1_1_37407,00.html. Accessed September 26, 2011.

33. Stock S, Drabik A, Büscher G, Graf C, Ulrich W, Gerber A, Lauterback KW, Lüngen M. German diabetes management programs improve quality of care and curb costs. *Health Aff.* 2010;29(12):2197–2205.

34. National Committee for Quality Improvement. The state of health care quality 2010. http://www.ncqa.org/portals/0/state%200f%20health%20care/2010/sohc%20 2010%20-%20fu112.pdf. Accessed September 10, 2011.

35. Morra D, Nicholson S, Levinson W, Gans DN, Hammons T, Casalino LP. U.S. physician practices versus Canadians: Spending nearly four times as much money interacting with payers. *Health Aff.* 2011;30(8):1443–1450.

36. Thomson S, Mossialos E. *Primary Care and Prescription Drugs: Coverage, Cost-Sharing, and Financial Protection in Six European Countries.* Commonwealth Fund; March 2010. http://www.commonwealthfund.org/~/media/Files/Publications/ Issue%20Brief/2010/Mar/1384_Thomson_primary_care_prescription_drugs_intl_ ib_325.pdf.

37. Andrews M. Value-based insurance design's pros and cons. *Washington Post,* November 29, 2010. http://www.washingtonpost.com/wp-dyn/content/ article/2010/11/29/AR2010112904751.html.

38. Fendrick AM, Chernew ME. Value-based insurance design: Aligning incentives to bridge the divide between quality improvement and cost containment. *Am J Managed Care.* 2006;12:SP5–SP10. http://www.sph.umich.edu/vbidcenter/publications/pdfs/ AJMC_06speclFendrick6p.pdf.

39. Project of the ABIM Foundation, ACP–ASIM Foundation, and European Federation of Internal Medicine. Medical professionalism in the new millennium: A physician charter. *Ann Intern Med.* 2002;136(3):243–246.

40. Project of the ABIM Foundation, ACP–ASIM Foundation, and European Federation of Internal Medicine. Medical professionalism in the new millennium: A physician charter. *Lancet.* 2002;359:520–522.

41. ABIM Foundation. Medical professionalism: Physician charter. http://www
.abimfoundation.org/Professionalism/Physician-Charter.aspx. Accessed August 14, 2011.

42. Chalkidou K. *Comparative Effectiveness Review within the U.K.'s National
Institute for Health and Clinical Excellence.* Commonwealth Fund; July 2009. http://www
.commonwealthfund.org/~/media/Files/Publications/Issue%20Brief/2009/Jul/
Chalkidou/1296_Chalkidou_UK_CER_issue_brief_717.pdf.

43. bpac[nz]. Best tests September 2011. http://bpac.org.nz/Public/home.asp. Accessed September 30, 2011.

44. Beecham L. NHS doctors in England face audit and annual appraisals. *BMJ.*
1999;319:1319.

45. General Medical Council. Revalidation, a statement of intent. October 2010.
http://www.gmc-uk.org/Revalidation_A_Statement_of_Intent_October_2010__
Final_version___web_version_.pdf_35982397.pdf.

46. General Medical Council. Revalidation. http://www.gmc-uk.org/doctors/
revalidation.asp. Accessed September 30, 2011.

47. Guterman S, Schoenbaum SC. Getting from here to there in payment reform:
Necessary practices and policies. *J Ambulatory Care Man.* 2010;33(1):53–57.

48. Bailit M, Hughes C. *Key Design Elements of Shared-Savings Payment
Arrangements.* Commonwealth Fund; August 2011. http://www.commonwealthfund
.org/~/media/Files/Publications/Issue%20Brief/2011/Aug/1539_Bailit_key_
design_elements_sharedsavings_ib_v2.pdf.

49. Cashin C, Chi Y-L. *Major Developments in Results-Based Financing (RBF) in
OECD Countries: Country Summaries and Mapping of RBF Programs: Australia: The
Practice Incentives Program (PIP).* World Bank; March 2011. http://www.rbfhealth
.org/rbfhealth/system/files/Case%20study%20Australia%20Practice%20Incentive%20
Program.pdf.

50. Gillam S. *Pay for Performance in UK General Practice—the Ambiguous Impact
of the Quality and Outcomes Framework.* National Quality Measures Clearinghouse,
Agency for Healthcare Research and Quality; March 2011. http://www.qualitymeasures
.ahrq.gov/expert/expert-commentary.aspx?id=25658. Accessed September 26, 2011.

51. Ferlie E, Shortell SM. Improving the quality of health care in the United Kingdom and the United States: A framework for change. *Milbank Q.* 2001;79(2):281–315.

52. Schoen C, Helms D, Folsom A. *Harnessing Health Care Markets for the Public
Interest: Insights for U.S. Health Reform from the German and Dutch Multipayer
Systems.* Commonwealth Fund and AcademyHealth; December 2009. http://www
.commonwealthfund.org/Publications/Fund-Reports/2009/Dec/Harnessing-Health-
Care-Markets-for-the-Public-Interest.aspx. Accessed September 26, 2011.

53. Schäfer W, Kroneman M, Boerma W, van den Berg M, Westert G, Devillé W,
van Ginneken E. The Netherlands health system review. *Health Systems in Transition.*
2010;12(1):1–267. http://www.nivel.nl/pdf/HIT-rapport-Netherland.pdf.

54. Petkantchin V. Health care reform in the Netherlands. Institut économique
Molinari's (IEM's) economic note. June 2010. http://www.institutmolinari.org/IMG/
pdf/note0610_en.pdf.

55. The NHS Plan: A plan for investment, a plan for reform. NHS white paper.

Presented to Parliament by the Secretary of State for Health by Command of Her Majesty, July 2000. http://webarchive.nationalarchives.gov.uk/20100407034821/http://www.dh.gov.uk/en/Publicationsandstatistics/Publications/PublicationsPolicyAndGuidance/DH_4002960. Accessed September 26, 2011.

56. Stevens S. Reform strategies for the English NHS. *Health Aff.* 2004;23(1):37–44.

57. Milburn A. Organizational and financial issues: 1999–2003. http://nhshistory.tryfan-online.co.uk/milburn.htm. Accessed September 30, 2011.

Conclusion

Future of Public Health

C. William Keck, F. Douglas Scutchfield,
and James W. Holsinger Jr.

It should be clear to readers that both the health of the public and the discipline and practice of public health in the United States are evolving rapidly. Measures of health status have, with some important exceptions, shown steady improvement since the beginning of the twentieth century. The practice of public health, broadly defined, is responsible for the majority of those gains. However, the contributions of public health have been largely unappreciated by the general public, and both the practice and the discipline have been overshadowed by the attention lavished on institutions and practitioners that provide personal medical care.

The last several decades, however, have witnessed a growing awareness both inside and outside the public health profession that achieving a higher level of community health will require more emphasis on health promotion and disease prevention and public policy initiatives that provide incentives to improve health outcomes. Important elements in creating this awareness and the accompanying movement for policy change have been the philosophic renaissance occurring in the public health profession since the late 1980s and the work of researchers that has made it clear that the improved application of preventive services and a community-based approach to affect the social determinants of health have the potential to improve health status. This is easier said than done, of course. Realizing this potential will require more resources for providing preventive services, improving the organization and delivery of individual and community preventive services, broadening the public health agenda to include the social determinants of health, melding medicine and public health in meaningful ways, and expanding research into public health services and systems. The Patient Protection and Affordable Care Act of 2010 (ACA) is supportive of these efforts; its provisions include incentives to improve the application of health promotion and disease prevention activities, large investments in public health practice, and support for the training of preventive medicine specialists, among other initiatives.[1] This concluding chapter reviews these elements, with particular attention paid to the systems changes that must occur in both public health and clinical medicine if citizens of the United States are to benefit from the knowledge we have and are developing about maintaining health. It also describes the particular challenges facing local health departments as they confront these new realities.

Evolution of the Public's Health

Health in the industrialized world has shown remarkable progress over the past 100 years. Gains in life expectancy and general health status in the United States have been part of this trend. In 1900 life expectancy at birth in the United States for all persons stood at 47.3 years (46.3 for men and 48.3 for women); by 2007 life expectancy for all persons had risen to 77.9 years (75.4 for men and 80.4 for women).[2] The infant mortality rate in 1900 was almost 100 infant deaths per 1,000 live births; by 2006 that number had dropped to 6.7.[3, 4] Similarly, death rates for all causes for all persons per 100,000 population declined from 1,719.0 in 1900 to 760.2 in 2007.[5-7] Many attribute these gains to the advances in clinical medicine that are so compellingly chronicled in the lay media. The fact is, however, that only about five of the approximately thirty years gained in life expectancy are the result of clinical curative interventions.[8]

Despite this good news, there is gathering evidence that all is not as well as it could be or should be in terms of U.S. health status. Even though it spends more than any other country on health care and has made significant gains in health over time, the United States currently ranks poorly on measures of health compared with the rest of the industrialized world, and it is losing ground. At the turn of the last century, when the World Health Organization ranked the effectiveness of the world's health systems, the United States was thirty-seventh—at the bottom of the industrialized nations.[9] The 2008 Robert Wood Johnson Foundation report *Overcoming Obstacles to Health* notes that the United States has slipped in both infant mortality rates—dropping from eighteenth in the world in 1980 to twenty-fifth in 2002—and life expectancy rates—dropping from fourteenth to twenty-third.[10] In addition, there are huge disparities in health among various U.S. subpopulations.[10] It is clear that high expenditures on health care have not brought concomitant gains in health to the average American.

Our failure to keep pace with the rest of the industrialized world in maintaining health, along with current trends in both the prevalence of precursors of chronic diseases and the prevalence of the diseases themselves, suggests that for the first time in our history, the next generation of Americans may be less healthy, on average, than their parents.[11] More than 1.5 million people in the United States die each year from chronic diseases (e.g., heart disease, cancer, stroke, chronic lung disease, diabetes), and many more suffer from the symptoms of these conditions. We know that health-destructive behaviors such as tobacco use, improper diet, and lack of physical activity are at the core of causation, and we are recognizing the strong correlation between sociocultural and physical environmental circumstances and the health "choices" made by individuals.[12, 13] In addition, the impact of poverty and inequality seems to go significantly beyond individual "choices" and thereby directly influences the health status of individuals. These "social determinants of health" affect disadvantaged populations disproportionately, and addressing them effectively will require a multisector societal approach that engages elements both inside and outside the health community.[14] The question is whether America's illness care industry, public health system, and other policy makers will be able to work together in the collaborative mode required to make significant future gains in health status. An important concern is the extent to which underresourced health departments can both maintain existing efforts and add new activities aimed at further improvements. They are, after all, the only agencies that have statutory responsibility for community health status. They are tasked with monitoring the community's health status, designing interventions aimed at correcting diagnosed health problems, implementing programs (often in partnership with others), and evaluating the impact of those interventions.

Evolution of the Discipline of Public Health

Organized public health departments began to appear in major cities along the East Coast during the late 1880s. After World War II, the nation's attention turned toward the development of acute care services, largely ignoring prevention and public health. Real expenditures on public health failed to keep pace with population growth, resulting in the parallel evolution of two separate disciplines—medicine and public health—with funding strongly and disproportionately supporting the former. With some variations and exceptions, that reality has persisted to the present, resulting in a public health infrastructure that is too weak to deliver the public health services that would permit a full achievement of positive health impacts if current knowledge could be generally applied.[15]

In more recent years, the emergence of new diseases (e.g., HIV/AIDS, SARS, drug-resistant tuberculosis), acts and threats of terrorism, and the relegation of "orphan" subjects (e.g., violence, genetics) to a broadening public health agenda have brought new attention to the discipline. But perhaps nothing stimulated the public health profession as much as the seminal study of the U.S. public health system performed by the Institute of Medicine (IOM) and described in its 1988 report *The Future of Public Health*.[16] The IOM's conclusion that the public health system was in disarray energized the public health community to remedy the problems outlined in that report.

Public Health's Philosophical Renaissance

Public health's efforts after the IOM report were stimulated by President Clinton's election in 1992 and his promise to pursue comprehensive health care reform. Past efforts at reform had paid scant attention to public health, and there was a general resolve among those in the public health profession that their field should be a strong component of this new initiative. The key to inclusion was to clearly define the role of public health in this country and to improve the general understanding of its needs and contributions. Using the IOM's findings and recommendations as a base, national public health professional associations, federal agencies, practitioners, and academics undertook to address the problems listed in the report. This collaboration resulted in a remarkable and continuing period that has witnessed notable progress in public health's role in improving population health status and the development and use of a variety of mechanisms to enhance the competence and effectiveness of its workforce (see box).

Over the past several decades, the profession has begun to clarify its role in terms that are understandable to the lay public, policy makers, and other members of the public health and clinical care systems. The three core functions of public health proposed by the IOM in 1988 were expanded into a list of ten essential services that communities must have in place in reasonable quantity and quality to reach the highest level of healthfulness (see box).[16, 17] It soon became clear that all these services could not be provided by even the best local health departments, so collaboration among and between clinical practitioners, health departments, nongovernmental organizations (NGOs), and other concerned parties would be required for overall community effectiveness. The Local Public Health System (LPHS) concept, as this came to be known, added weight to the idea that the United States could benefit from a better merging of medicine, public health, and the organizations and agencies that contribute to the mission of public health: "creating conditions in which people can be healthy."[18] From the list of essential services, a set of national public health performance standards was developed to allow communities to

Major Accomplishments of the Past Two Decades

- IOM's identification of the core functions of public health:
  - Assessment
  - Policy development
  - Assurance[16]
- Identification of the ten essential public health services[17]
- Creation of the concept of the Local Public Health System (LPHS), illustrating the need for all health-related entities in a community to collaborate so that the community can reach the maximum level of healthfulness[18]
- National public health performance standards for state and local health departments and local public health governance organizations[19]
- Workforce skill enhancement:
  - Core competencies for public health professionals[20]
  - National and state public health leadership institutes[21]
  - Steady increase in the number of schools of public health and MPH degree programs[22]
  - Teaching of public health at the undergraduate level[23]
  - Teaching of public health in medical schools[24]
  - Renewed support for the training of specialists in preventive medicine[1]
- Process to credential public health professionals[25]
- Public health code of ethics[26]
- Process to accredit local and state health departments using national standards[27]
- Creation of guidelines for community preventive services[29]
- Public health services and systems research agenda with practice-based research networks[30]

quantify their ability to deliver those essential services, improve their quality, and make the work of public health both accountable and transparent.[19]

A concomitant concern was how to address the workforce and organizational capacity of public health. Core competencies for public health workers were developed and adopted,[20] and state and national public health leadership institutes were created to identify tomorrow's likely public health leaders and better equip them for leadership.[21] The number of schools of public health and master's of public health (MPH) degree programs has been steadily increasing,[22] and a growing number of colleges and universities now offer

The Ten Essential Services

1. Monitor health status to identify community health problems.
2. Diagnose and investigate health problems and health hazards in the community.
3. Inform, educate, and empower people about health issues.
4. Mobilize community partnerships to identify and solve health problems.
5. Develop policies and plans that support individual and community health efforts.
6. Enforce laws and regulations that protect health and ensure safety.
7. Link people to needed personal health services and ensure the provision of health care when otherwise unavailable.
8. Assure a competent public health and personal health care workforce.
9. Evaluate effectiveness, accessibility, and quality of personal and population-based health services.
10. Research for new insights and innovative solutions to health problems.[17]

undergraduate public health courses.[23] Expanding and improving the teaching of public health in medical schools has been promoted by the Association of American Medical Colleges and the Centers for Disease Control and Prevention (CDC),[24] and the ACA contains provisions to support the training of specialists in preventive medicine.[1] A voluntary certification process has been implemented to ensure that public health workers achieve a minimum level of competence,[25] and a new code of public health ethics has been developed to guide ethical action.[26] At the same time, a process to accredit local health departments is in the early stages of implementation.[27] This is being assisted in sixteen states by the Robert Wood Johnson's Multistate Learning Collaborative, which focuses on applying quality improvement methods in local and state health departments while preparing them for national voluntary accreditation.[28] Public health is no longer in the position of being the only major health profession without a process to certify its practitioners or accredit its agencies.

In general, the effectiveness of public health interventions had not been subjected to the same scientific rigor as clinical interventions, but this is changing. The Task Force on Community Preventive Services is now bringing rigor to public health practices,[29] and the Center for Public Health Services and Systems Research is focusing attention on how best to provide a public health infrastructure to implement those practices.[30] These activities demonstrate that public health is in the midst of a true renaissance in its underlying philosophy, its role, the quality of its workforce and institutions, and its effectiveness. Unfortunately, that renaissance has not significantly affected the organization and funding of public health activities. Little progress has been made in depoliticizing local and state health departments, repairing and maintaining a frayed public health infrastructure, and addressing the extremely wide variation in sophistication and capacity among health departments across the country.

Public Health Organization and Funding

Despite the growing unity of thought about public health's core functions and essential services and its efforts to improve the quality of its workforce, the question remains: do local and state health departments actually have the capability to carry out the tasks that are currently required and will likely be required in the future? Regrettably, there are still wide gaps between the public health taught in academia and that practiced in the community. There is great variability in structure, governance, and capacity among health departments at the local and state levels. Surveys of the country's approximately 3,000 local health departments (LHDs) performed by the National Association of County and City Health Officials (NACCHO) over time clearly illustrate the differences in governance structure, jurisdictional type, governing body, size, source and amount of revenue, and services offered.[31] There are limited means to judge the capacity of LHDs, but it is instructive to note that these agencies serve populations ranging from approximately 10 million in Los Angeles County to communities as small as 1,000 people. As a matter of fact, the majority of LHDs serve relatively small populations. In 2010, 63 percent of the nation's LHDs served communities with fewer than 50,000 residents, and 42 percent served those with less than 25,000 residents. Departments serving populations of 10,000 to 25,000 people had a median of nine full-time staff members (expressed as full-time equivalents [FTEs]), those serving populations of 50,000 to 100,000 had thirty FTEs, and those serving 100,000 to 500,000 had eighty-three FTEs.[31] Departmental size does not necessarily correlate with the quality of services provided, of course; there are many excellent small health departments. Size does correlate with capacity, however, and larger health departments are more likely to have a broader range of skilled professionals with higher levels of specialized skills (e.g., physicians, epidemiologists, environmental health scientists, information specialists). This would increase the department's potential to effectively pursue public health's assessment, policy development, and assurance functions.[32] There is now evidence that larger departments serving populations up to 500,000 do perform better, so size *does* matter.[33] Such variability is problematic from the perspective of the equitable distribution of effective services among the entire U.S. population. It is a mistake to think of public health in this country as a "system": each state and territory is a separate governmental entity, and most LHDs are locally governed, even though in some states they are part of the state health department. Needless to say, there is no evidence suggesting which organizational pattern is better—an indication of how difficult it is in a large democracy with strong traditions of home rule to develop consistency of thought and action. In many locations, LHDs are simply too small and too resource poor to carry out all the activities expected of them, and they often rely on grant dollars and the rules that accompany them to create some unity of approach across health department jurisdictions. One helpful result of the 2008–2011 economic slowdown is that it encouraged some LHDs to collaborate and cooperate with other small adjoining health departments in an effort to diminish costs and expand impact.[34]

The last decade has been something of a boom and bust cycle in terms of funding for state and local health departments. At the end of the twentieth century, growing concern about terrorism and the potential use of biological weapons highlighted the need to improve an inadequate public health infrastructure.[35] As a result, the CDC instituted cooperative agreements for public health emergency preparedness to provide funding and technical assistance to selected state and local health departments to support the unified development of emergency response plans.[36] The 2001 terrorist attacks in the United States dramatically renewed the country's interest in preventing and, if necessary, responding to emergencies of all kinds, especially terrorism. Public health, emergency management, and medical, fire, and police officials had to learn to communicate and cooperate in new ways, and federal money was quickly appropriated to improve preparedness and emergency response capabilities. Suddenly, long-neglected infrastructure, particularly in public health, received new attention and resources. By fiscal year 2007, more than $5 billion had been distributed to sixty-two state, local, territorial, and tribal health departments, although amounts have been declining annually since 2005.[36] NACCHO reported in 2008 that LHDs had shown steady improvement in all-hazards emergency response, mass prophylaxis, and communication plans; compliance with incident command guidelines; workforce training; National Incident Management System (NIMS) compliance; and participation in emergency response drills.[37]

In many LHDs, some core functions, such as disease surveillance and epidemiologic analysis, were also strengthened by the technical assistance and funding support for all-hazards preparedness. However, serious decreases in funding, especially for areas unrelated to emergency preparedness, became the norm for both state and local health departments when the severe economic recession began at the end of 2007. By January 2012, about 57 percent of LHDs had been forced to cut core public health programs such as maternal and child health, population-based primary prevention, environmental health, clinical health services, and immunizations. A NACCHO survey revealed that between 2008 and 2012, about 39,600 public health jobs were lost to layoffs or attrition.[38] A 2010 NACCHO survey revealed that by June of that year an additional 18,000 public health workers had their hours reduced directly or through mandatory furloughs. This prompted NACCHO to warn that continued budget cuts "undermine the ability of LHDs to protect the public from preventable diseases, environmental hazards, and other threats to public health."[39] This concern was echoed by the Association of State and Territorial Health Officials, which noted that the fiscal crisis was affecting state and territorial health agencies in similar ways. About 17,800 state jobs were lost during this period, and more were expected to disappear when federal funding through the American Recovery and Reinvestment Act of 2009 disappeared in fiscal year 2012. The result to date has been a combined loss of 57,400 jobs in state and local health departments and significant cuts to core public health programs in many states.[40, 41]

Challenges and Opportunities

The press of current events, along with the guidance and challenges offered by the IOM's 1988 report,[16] provided the impetus at the end of the last century to better define the role and practice of public health, improve its capacity, and better train its workers. About fifteen years later, much had changed in public health practice and the population demographics affecting it, and the IOM received funding from a variety of federal governmental agencies to convene the Committee on Assuring the Health of the Public in the 21st Century to create a framework for ensuring future population health in the United States; its report was published in 2003.[18] More recently, the Robert Wood Johnson Foundation supported the work of the IOM Committee on Public Health Strategies to Improve Health by examining measurement, the law, and funding in public health (discussed later). These reports, as well as changes in the understanding of health precursors and shifts in organization and funding environments, are coalescing to identify both challenges and opportunities for public health, especially for state and local health departments.

The Future of the Public's Health

The IOM Committee on Assuring the Health of the Public in the 21st Century had a broader charge than the committee that published the 1988 report. Whereas the earlier work focused principally on state and local health departments—governmental public health agencies—the later effort recognized that improving health required the participation of the entire LPHS—"a complex network of individuals and organizations that, when working together, can represent what we as a society do collectively to assure the conditions in which people can be healthy."[18] In addition to the governmental public health infrastructure, this committee looked at the community, the health care delivery system, employers, the media, and academia. It made recommendations for both the governmental public health infrastructure and other community entities (see boxes).

IOM Recommendations for the
Governmental Public Health Infrastructure

- Develop a framework and recommendations for state public health law reform to meet modern scientific and legal standards and foster greater consistency across states.
- Develop strategies to ensure that public health workers demonstrate mastery of the core public health competencies.
- Assess periodically the preparedness of the public health workforce, and document and fund necessary training.
- Give high priority to leadership training, support, and development for public health professionals.
- Develop a system of public health workforce credentialing.
- Improve the use of existing and emerging communication tools.
- Facilitate the development of the national health information infrastructure.
- Assess and report on the state of the nation's governmental public health infrastructure and its capacity to provide essential services.
- Evaluate the status of the nation's public health laboratory system.
- Develop a comprehensive investment plan for a strong national governmental public health infrastructure.
- Experiment with clustering or consolidating categorical grants.
- Consider the usefulness of an accreditation system for improving and building state and local health department capacities.
- Develop a research agenda and estimate the funding needed to build

the evidence base required to guide policy making for public health practice.

- Review the regulatory authority of Department of Health and Human Services (DHHS) agencies with health-related responsibilities to reduce overlap and inconsistencies and ensure good coordination within DHHS and with state and local health departments.
- Establish a National Public Health Council consisting of the secretary of DHHS and state health commissioners to advise the secretary and provide a forum to oversee the development of an incentive-based federal- and state-funded system to sustain a governmental public health infrastructure capable of assuring the delivery of essential services.[18]

IOM Recommendations for Others

- LHDs should work with other community groups to inventory resources, assess needs, formulate collaborative responses, and evaluate outcomes of efforts to improve community health and eliminate health disparities.
- Comprehensive and affordable health care should be available to each U.S. resident.
- Effective preventive services, as well as oral health, mental health, and substance abuse treatment, should be available to all.
- The corporate community and public health agencies should collaborate in workplace health promotion and disease and injury prevention programs.
- Public health professionals and media outlets should work together to enhance and improve public service announcements and to develop an evidence base on the media's influence on health knowledge and behavior and on the promotion of healthy public policy.
- Prevention research should be enhanced and should focus on improving population health.[18]

Many of the recommendations made by the IOM committee in 2003 either are under development or were included in the ACA passed by Congress in 2010.[1] Processes for worker certification and agency accreditation are now in place and can be expected to expand over time. A network of leadership institutes is focusing on expanding the competencies of public health workers.[21] A Public Health Services and Systems Research Center has been established,[26] and public health practice-based research networks are in place and likely to grow.[42]

The ACA addresses issues such as expanded access to health care, availability of prevention services, training of preventive medicine specialists, ongoing funding for public health infrastructure, workplace health, and collaborative networks within communities.[1] These elements will all be important as the discipline of public health evolves and in the collaborative efforts of components of the LPHS.

For the Public's Health

In 2009 the Robert Wood Johnson Foundation provided support for the IOM to convene a "Committee on Public Health Strategies to Improve Health" to examine three public health–related topics: measurement, the law, and funding. The committee is exploring these topics in the context of current challenges and opportunities inherent in a reformed health system, with the goal of influencing the work of the LPHS in the second decade of the twenty-first century and beyond. In other words, now that the ACA is law, what can be done to help all elements of the LPHS improve population health? The three reports are *For the Public's Health: The Role of Measurement in Action and Accountability*,[43] *For the Public's Health: Revitalizing Law and Policy to Meet New Challenges*,[44] and *For the Public's Health: Investing in a Healthier Future*.[45] In the words of the authors of the first report:

> The expected reform of the clinical care delivery system and the committee's understanding of the centrality of socio-environmental determinants of health led it to view measures of health outcomes . . . as serving three primary functions:
>
> • To provide transparent and easily understood information to members of communities and the public and private entities that serve them about health and the stakeholders that influence it locally and nationally.
> • To galvanize and promote participation and responsibility on the part of the public and institutional stakeholders (business, employers, community members, and others) that have roles to play in improving population health.

- To foster greater accountability for performance in health improvement on the part of government health agencies, other government entities whose portfolios have direct bearing on the health of Americans, and private-sector and nonprofit-sector contributors to the health system.[43]

The committee advocates a transformation of the national data system to better track health and its determinants in a fashion that can be generally understood and utilized to both stimulate positive action and evaluate outcomes. It envisions a reinvigorated approach to improving health that diminishes competition among clinical providers and refocuses components of the LPHS on collaboration to improve health status—a significant change from most current practices.

The committee responsible for the second report believes that it is critical to examine the role and usefulness of laws and public policies more broadly, both inside and outside the health sector, in an effort to improve population health. Its recommendations apply to three major areas:

- Laws and public policies that pertain to population health should be systematically reviewed and revised, given the enormous transformations in the practice, context, science, and goals of public health agencies and changes in society as a whole.
- Government agencies should familiarize themselves with the toolbox of public health legal and policy interventions at their disposal.
- Government and private-sector stakeholders should explore and embrace a "health in all policies" approach for its synergistic potential.[44]

The same theme of a broad societal approach to improving health persists in the final report on financing public health services. Recommendations made by the committee focus on two major areas: insufficient funding levels for public health services and programs, and dysfunction in how the public health infrastructure is funded, organized, and equipped to use its funding.[45]

If successful, these recommendations and subsequent actions should shift the public policy debate in the United States away from arguments about power and money and more toward what should be done to improve health status. These trends have significant implications for the future of state and local health departments.

Mission Creep

Public health's origins in the United States are rooted in the struggle to control communicable diseases. Initial efforts focused on environmental issues, such as crowding and safe food and water. As time passed and more effective tools were developed, the mission of public health was steadily broadened to include such things as maternal and child health and the distribution of vaccines. When chronic diseases became the major threat to Americans' health in the middle of the twentieth century, this created an impetus to address their causes from a population perspective; then the so-called "War on Poverty" in the 1960s added a variety of social issues to public health's mission.[15] Health departments are the only entities with statutory and fiduciary responsibility for community health status, so it is not surprising that expectations of these departments broaden as awareness and needs dictate. This "mission creep" is ongoing and occurs in three major categories: extension of current activities, default, and science.

Extension of current activities

Public health departments' historical responsibility for infectious disease surveillance and response meant their immediate involvement in such threats as emerging infections (HIV/AIDS, SARS, drug-resistant tuberculosis) and bioterrorism. Likewise, new programs to control air pollutants and other environmental hazards are based on a long and broad history of involvement in environmental control programs.

Default

For many years, health departments have provided a medical care safety net for conditions and populations that fell through the wide cracks in the U.S. health care industry. Sexually transmitted disease and tuberculosis clinics were natural extensions of public health's communicable disease control responsibility, but prenatal care, well-child care, and the general primary care offered by some health departments are in place only because certain populations lacked access to private health services. The population focus of public health makes it the obvious place to turn to address health disparities among subpopulations or the implications of new knowledge about genomics.

Science

Ensuring that scientific discoveries relevant to population health are available to all has long been at the core of public health practice. The Task Force on Community Preventive Services has increased awareness of the effectiveness of many core public health activities and clarified which activities should be continued and strengthened and which have little or no data to support their use.[29] The work of the Council on Linkages between Public Health Academia and Practice[46] and the Center for Public Health Services and Systems Research[30] has brought additional attention to the need for research on population health issues and methods of improving health status.

As we achieve a better understanding of the factors underlying the development of chronic diseases, and as the U.S. health status continues to decrease, it is clear that improving health in the United States will require substantial changes in the way clinical care and public health services are delivered.

Social Determinants of Health

Important work is being done to better understand the social determinants of health. Chapter 1 reviews the current understanding of the interrelationships among people's health, education, occupation, income, housing, racial and ethnic background, and other socioecological factors. Our focus on using the existing illness care industry to improve the overall health of the population and to reduce the rather substantial racial, ethnic, and geographic disparities has had limited effect.[47] The Robert Wood Johnson Foundation sponsored a commission made up of diverse individuals in terms of discipline, experience, and political ideology and asked them to make recommendations for population health improvement. They concluded: "Although medical care is important, our reviews of research and the hearings we've held have led us to conclude that building a healthier America will hinge largely on what we do beyond the health care system. It means changing policies that influence economic opportunity, early childhood development, schools, housing, the workplace, community design and nutrition, so that all Americans can live, work, play, and learn in environments that protect and actively promote health."[48] Or, as more strongly put by Marmot and Bell: "Social injustice is killing people on a grand scale"; "the poor health of the poor, the social gradient in health within countries, and the marked health inequalities between countries are caused by the unequal distribution of power, income, goods, and services, globally and nationally, the consequent unfairness in the immediate, visible circumstances of people's lives. . . . This unequal distribution of health damaging experience . . . is the result of a toxic combination of poor social policies and programmes, unfair economic arrangements and bad politics."[14] Health departments, as the community's agent for dealing with the risk factors responsible for poor health, must accept this new and perplexing mission: how to address issues responsible for poor health status that are outside both the usual health sphere and the traditional purview of the health department. Some may see such intervention by the health department as "meddling" in areas that are not its concern.

The Patient Protection and Affordable Care Act

In the United States, major public policy discussions at the national level have rarely been primarily about improving health. Rather, the focus has been predominantly on power and money—who pays for what clinical services, and how much. The ACA, signed into law by President Obama in March 2010, certainly spends a great deal of ink on payment structures for clinical services, but it also focuses on health promotion, disease prevention, wellness, and the improvement of health outcomes. Its provisions include the establishment of a National Prevention, Health Promotion, and Public Health Council to bring cabinet department secretaries together under the auspices of the surgeon general to determine how to improve the health impact of programs and policies in areas of government that are not explicitly concerned with health. Another task of the council is to develop a national prevention and health promotion strategy, and the ACA created a Prevention and Wellness Trust Fund to support the development of measureable goals for such a strategy.[1] The trust fund's first report, which was made public in June 2011, describes the overarching goal of the national prevention strategy: to increase the number of Americans who are healthy at every stage of life. The report also provides four evidence-based strategic directions that will require the active engagement of all sectors of society to achieve: (1) build healthy and safe community environments, (2) expand quality preventive services in both clinical and community settings, (3) empower people to make healthy choices, and (4) eliminate health disparities.[49]

The act also expands the work of the Task Force on Community Preventive Services and provides $15 billion over ten years to fund public health infrastructure and workforce initiatives—the largest single investment in the public health system ever made in the United States. There are also provisions that foster the type of partnerships required to address health holistically, including incentives for clinical settings to collaborate with community-based agencies to improve health outcomes.[1] Despite the act's admitted problems, it is a remarkable document that recognizes the importance of changing the way health is approached in the United States if we are to achieve more efficient health services and improved health outcomes.

Communication Infrastructure

The rapid evolution of electronic infrastructure has transformed modern society. Systems related to health have often been slow to adopt new technologies, but that is rapidly changing. The growing capacity to store, analyze, and transmit information allows social, behavioral, and medical data to be combined to help detect disease before it manifests and to support both treatment and health promotion. Mobile computer and Internet platforms allow the coordination of health services by clinical and public health providers, and they empower consumers to manage their own health, all informed by data on the health of the general population or specific population subgroups.[50]

In an effort to use health information technology (HIT) to improve health outcomes and reduce the costs of health care, the federal government's HIT strategic plan supports activities that improve individual patient care and encourage population health research and practice. Both efforts will require access to a national health information infrastructure that enables the sharing of electronic health information.[51] Substantial financial support will be required, and initial steps to provide it have been taken through the Health Information Technology for Economic and Clinical Health Act, part of the American Recovery and Reinvestment Act of 2009 and the ACA. There are exciting opportunities here for both the clinical and the public health components of the LPHS to make significant strides in HIT. Given the growth of hand-held computing and communication technologies available to the average consumer, the impact is likely to be limited only by what can be imagined.

Public Health's Future

The second decade of the twenty-first century is an exciting but challenging time to be a public health practitioner. The profession has redefined and reinvigorated itself in many ways and has come to the understanding that it must collaborate directly and effectively with other agencies, institutions, and individuals to fulfill its mission. Perhaps for the first time since the early decades of the twentieth century, national policy makers recognize the importance of public health and prevention in the struggle to improve health status, and resources have been directed or promised to local public health agencies and others to improve services and support research. So, in this evolving world, what would a successful LPHS look like? To answer that question, we examine the effective health department of the future, as well as the interaction of that entity with other members of the LPHS.

The local health department

One of the few constants in public health practice is that change is ongoing and increasingly rapid. The public health department's mission continues to expand while resources tend to diminish. New responsibilities require new skills and innovative leaders who are willing to reach out and partner with others. Electronic technology must be harnessed to improve health surveillance, communication, and evaluation activities. The number of credentialed public health workers can be expected to increase, and as the public becomes increasingly aware of health department activities, it will expect sufficient capacity and quality for agency accreditation. Currency in workforce development and recruitment, as well as participation in community-based research, will require connections with academic institutions. Effectiveness will be predicated, at least in part, on measurable improvements in community health status over time, and health departments are likely to be held accountable for those improvements.

The effective health department of the future will be aware of these currents of change and will demonstrate the capacity and flexibility to adjust existing activities and develop new ones to ensure effectiveness. The public health department must be the health intelligence center of its community. It should have the surveillance and community assessment capacity to be the source of epidemiologically based thinking and analysis of the community's approach to health issues, and it should facilitate the community's response to identified health problems. Part of that facilitation involves the ability to either deliver or broker the delivery of services required by its constituent populations. Given the importance of the social determinants of health, the health department (along with others) must be a strong participant in the public policy arena as well. Health outcomes should be used as the definitive measure of effectiveness.[52]

The capacity of a health department to work effectively, now and in the future, depends on many factors, and size is one of them.[33] The range of skills and activities required will vary somewhat by community (large or small, rich or poor, healthy or unhealthy), but many LHDs are too small to provide all the essential public health services. How small is too small cannot be clearly stated at this point, although as the agency accreditation process proceeds, more information about the relationship between department size and the ability to achieve accreditation—a measure of effectiveness—should emerge. Certainly, a department will function best when its geographic boundaries of authority make sense to its constituents, funding is relatively stable, and the tax base is sufficient to provide the local share of resources required to accomplish at least the core functions of public health. The fact that some small health departments have merged with others or are considering sharing agreements or memos of understanding suggests that this is a response to economic realities, to the existence of national performance standards against which capacity and effectiveness can be measured, and to the push for agency accreditation. Whether these forces continue to stimulate efforts to create a critical mass of resources to improve capacity remains to be seen, but their existence has helped move the relatively disparate world of 3,000 locally governed health departments closer to a national system than ever before. Currently, there are uniform national expectations with regard to capacity and performance that can be followed voluntarily, and it is possible that pressure will grow for every health department to participate in the national voluntary accreditation effort.

In addition to staff size and resources, governance structure is important. Effective health departments will have a governance structure that clearly delegates policy-making decisions to the board of health (or other governing body) and administrative functions to the director of the department. Moreover, the department's primary concern must be the description and solution of public health problems in the constituent community, rather than the political correctness of its activities. There is evidence that having a policy-making board of health improves performance.[53] While the many nuances of governance and its influence on effectiveness are not understood, it is an area that merits attention as health departments strive for improved quality.

The electronic revolution is a classic mixture of challenges and opportunities for public health departments. Effectiveness will require high-speed Internet connections for most, if not all, employees and the capacity to sort through and correctly interpret relevant information and respond appropriately. Disease surveillance systems must be fine-tuned, and the capacity to communicate with other LPHS members must be highly functional. The ability to interact with constituents in ways that respond to requests for assistance and inform individuals how to maintain or improve their health is also important. Perhaps the most difficult and expensive undertaking in this area will be the development of electronic health records. The ACA, in a quest for improved efficiency and effectiveness in clinical settings, provides strong incentives for their use. This is especially true for participants in accountable care organizations (ACOs), as defined in the act. Health departments are not listed as required partners in forming ACOs, but they may find it advantageous to either join an ACO or partner with one in providing some elements of patient care. Such departments will almost certainly need electronic health records that are compatible with those of existing and potential partners.

The United States is one of the most culturally diverse nations on earth. A health department that is not culturally sensitive and competent will be limited in its effectiveness as it encourages and enables citizens to take care of their own health and to participate in decision making related to individual as well as community health needs, and as it assesses the impact of programs and services designed to improve community health. One element of cultural competency is to ensure that minority groups are represented in the public health workforce.

The goal of every citizen being served by a competent public health agency will not become a reality in the absence of strong and effective agency leadership. Effective health departments will have leaders who exhibit commitment, charisma, and drive and who embrace collective action, community empowerment, consumer advocacy, and egalitarianism.[54] These latter qualities will be increasingly important as health departments move into multiple partnerships to develop shared services and affect the social determinants of health.

Working within the local public health system

LHDs are accountable for the mission of public health—that is, "creating conditions in which people can be healthy"—but this mission is shared with a number of other community organizations and institutions.[16] No matter how effective an LHD is, it probably will not have all the resources needed to ameliorate all unhealthful conditions and provide all the health promotion and disease prevention services a population needs. This is especially true in an environment of diminishing resources in the public sector (with the notable exception of the promise of ACA funding), coupled with a growing body of knowledge identifying "upstream" antecedents to disease that have traditionally not been the purview of health departments or other health-related institutions.[12, 55] This expansion of responsibility, including the need to develop new approaches to impact the social determinants of health, suggests that successful partnering with others is both an economic and a programmatic necessity.

The effective health department of the future will therefore be the coordinator of a community-wide effort to develop and implement a broad health promotion strategy. This will, of necessity, include many sectors of society (e.g., education, business, clinical practitioners, NGOs concerned with health, public health, general government, citizens groups) in the effort to create conditions that support sustainable health improvements.[56] The ACA's expanded public health finding and requirement for the development of ACOs will create new opportunities for participation and collaboration in expanding the ACO idea to the concept of the accountable care community (ACC)—an initiative to integrate community assets into a framework of shared responsibility for improvement in community health.[57] This is a significant paradigm shift and is daunting to contemplate. A stepwise approach to establishing these new relationships may be easier than trying to do so "all at once."

Collaborating on clinical and community preventive measures

Initiatives that involve behavior modification are generally not well handled in clinical practice settings. Programs for smoking cessation and substance abuse (alcohol and other drugs), along with counseling about diet and exercise, may be available in some communities through LHDs or nongovernmental organizations such as the American Heart Association, American Cancer Society, American Lung Association, Kidney Foundation, and Diabetes Association. It is unusual, however, for these programs to be part of the mainstream of patient care, consistently available, and of uniformly high quality. Given today's focus on prevention and wellness, it may be time to form new alliances among clinical care settings, governmental organizations, and NGOs and pool their resources to create referral centers that combine science-supported individual patient care with community-based programs (see box). These types of collaboration would set the stage for the next step—moving upstream to address the social determinants of health.

Behavioral Change Centers

In a new medical care–public health collaborative system, a community's hospitals, LHDs, and NGOs interested in health behaviors (e.g., smoking cessation, weight reduction, exercise counseling) could pool their resources to create a year-round, scientifically sound program that offers behavior change support services to individuals. The services provided would emphasize the clinical preventive services in clinical care settings, and the professional relationships developed would set the stage for coordinated community preventive services.

In practice, a physician would make an appointment at the behavioral change center for her patient and send a formal request for consultation and evaluation, just as she would if she wanted a surgical opinion. Once the patient is enrolled, progress notes will be shared with the referring physician. That way, when the doctor sees her patient again, she will be able to encourage her efforts to stop smoking or reinforce the need to apply herself to weight loss and exercise.

Physicians would likely be pleased with such a new community resource. With its assistance, they would be able to have a greater impact on the health of their patients, and it would make them more aware of the need to support health-related policy decisions at the community level.

Moving upstream

The challenges and opportunities for LHDs in galvanizing communities to address the early antecedents of disease are substantial. To be an effective galvanizer of community action, the department will need a community diagnosis that provides the database to support the necessity for action, the leadership capacity to both convene the individuals required for success and organize the community's response, and the capacity to measure programmatic impact. The quest for success will involve venturing into policy arenas where health voices have not been heard previously (e.g., planning and zoning, development). To help assess issues' and policies' likely impact on health before final decisions are made, health departments may consider the relatively new health impact assessment (HIA) tool.[55, 58, 59] Linkages with academic institutions, when available, could prove helpful in completing HIAs, developing intervention strategies, and assessing outcomes.

The second decade of the twenty-first century is an extraordinary time for the public health profession. Its role in shaping improvements in health status has never been clearer, and national public policy is increasingly synchronous with that role. Success will require embracing the paradigm shift presented by the need to address the social determinants of health while maintaining other basic services, dealing with resource limitations, and developing the necessary new partnerships. If public health can break out of old molds and old modes of operation, there is every reason to expect that public health will continue to fulfill its mission to improve community health status.

Notes

1. Patient Protection and Affordable Care Act (HR 3590). March 23, 2010. https://www.annualmedicalreport.com/text-of-health-care-bill-patient-protection-and-affordable-care-act-hr-3590-text-of-bill.

2. National Center for Health Statistics. Health, United States, 2010. Table 22. http://www.cdc.gov/nchs/data/hus/hus10.pdf#listtables. Accessed May 16, 2011.

3. Centers for Disease Control and Prevention. Achievements in public health, 1900–1999: Healthier mothers and babies. *MMWR Morb Mortal Wkly Rep.* 1999;48(38):849–858.   http://www.cdc.gov/mmwr/preview/mmwrhtml/mm4838a2.htm#fig1. Accessed May 17, 2011.

4. National Center for Health Statistics. Health, United States, 2010. Table 15. http://www.cdc.gov/nchs/data/hus/hus10.pdf#listtables. Accessed May 16, 2011.

5. National Center for Health Statistics. Historical data. http://www.cdc.gov/nchs/data/dvs/hist290_0039.pdf. Accessed May 17, 2011.

6. National Center for Health Statistics. Historical data. http://www.cdc.gov/nchs/data/dvs/mx194049.pdf. Accessed May 17, 2011.

7. National Center for Health Statistics. Health, United States, 2010. Table 29. http://www.cdc.gov/nchs/data/hus/hus10.pdf#listtables. Accessed May 16, 2011.

8. Bunker JP, Frazier HS, Mosteller F. Improving health: Measuring effects of medical care. *Milbank Q.* 1994;72(2):225–258.

9. World Health Organization. *World Health Report. 1997. Ranking of the World's Health Systems.* http://www.photius.com/rankings/healthranks/html. Accessed May 16, 2011.

10. Robert Wood Johnson Foundation. *Overcoming Obstacles to Health: Report from the Robert Wood Johnson Foundation to the Commission to Build a Healthier America.* Princeton, NJ: Robert Wood Johnson Foundation; 2008.

11. Carmona RH. The growing epidemic of childhood obesity. Testimony before the U.S. Senate Committee on Commerce, Science, and Transportation, Subcommittee on Competition, Infrastructure, and Foreign Commerce. March 2, 2004. http://www.surgeongeneral.gov/news/testimony/childobesity03022004.html. Accessed September 14, 2011.

12. Braveman PA, Egerter SA, Mockenhaupt RE. Broadening the focus: The need to address the social determinants of health. *Am J Prev Med.* 2011;40(1 Suppl 1):S4–S18.

13. Woolf SH, Dekker MM, Byrne FR, Miller WD. Citizen-centered health promotion: Building collaborations to facilitate healthy living. *Am J Prev Med.* 2011;40(1 Suppl 1):S38–S47.

14. Marmot MG, Bell RG. Improving health: Social determinants and personal choice. *Am J Prev Med.* 2011;40(1 Suppl 1):S73–S77.

15. Fee E. History and development of public health. In: Scutchfield FD, Keck CW, eds. *Principles of Public Health Practice.* 3rd ed. Clifton Park, NY: Delmar Cengage Learning; 2009.

16. Institute of Medicine, Committee for the Study of the Future of Public Health. *The Future of Public Health.* Washington, DC: National Academies Press; 1988.

17. Public Health Functions Steering Committee. Public health in America. 1994. http://www.health.gov/phfunctions/public.html. Accessed May 19, 2011.

18. Institute of Medicine, Committee on Assuring the Health of the Public in the 21st Century. *The Future of the Public's Health in the 21st Century.* Washington, DC: National Academies Press; 2003.

19. Centers for Disease Control and Prevention. Assessment instruments 2008 to present. http://www.cdc.gov/nphpsp/theInstruments.html. Accessed May 19, 2011.

20. Council on Linkages between Public Health Academia and Practice. Core competencies for public health professionals. 2010. http://www.phf.org/resourcestools/Pages/Core_Public_Health_Competencies.aspx. Accessed May 19, 2011.

21. National Network of Public Health Institutes. http://www.nnphi.org/. Accessed May 19, 2011.

22. By the end of 2010, the Council on Education for Public Health (CEPH) was accrediting forty-eight schools of public health (SPHs) and eighty-three programs of public health (PHPs). Between 1990 and 2000, twelve new SPHs and forty-nine new

PHPs were accredited. In 2011 CEPH had three new formal applications for accreditation from SPHs and twenty-eight from PHPs. Many other schools and programs are in development. Personal communication, Laura Razor, executive director, CEPH, July 8, 2011.

23. Riegelman RK, Albertine S. Undergraduate public health at 4-year institutions: It's here to stay. *Am J Prev Med.* 2011;40(2):226–231.

24. Patients and populations: Public health in medical education. *Am J Prev Med.* 2011;41(3 Suppl):S145–S318.

25. National Board of Public Health Examiners. http://www.publichealthexam.org/. Accessed May 20, 2011.

26. Thomas JC, Sage M, Dillenberg J, Guillory J. A code of ethics for public health. *Am J Public Health.* 2002;92(7):1057–1059. http://www.ncbi.nlm.nih.gov/pmc/articles/PMC1447186/. Accessed May 19, 2011.

27. Public Health Accreditation Board. http://www.phaboard.org/. Accessed May 20, 2011.

28. Joly BM, Shaler G, Booth M, Conway A, Mittal P. Evaluating the multi-state learning collaborative. *J Public Health Manage Pract.* 2010;16(1):61–66.

29. Task Force on Community Preventive Services. *The Guide to Community Preventive Services.* New York: Oxford University Press; 2005. http://www.thecommunityguide.org/library/book/index.html. Accessed May 19, 2011.

30. Center for Public Health Services and Systems Research, University of Kentucky. http://www.publichealthsystems.org/cphssr. Accessed May 20, 2011.

31. National Association of County and City Health Officials. *National Profile of Local Health Departments.* Washington, DC: NACCHO; 2010.

32. Leep CJ, Gorenflo G, Libbey PM. The local health department. In: Scutchfield FD, Keck CW, eds. *Principles of Public Health Practice.* 3rd ed. Clifton Park, NY: Delmar Cengage Learning; 2009.

33. Mays GP, Smith SA. Geographic variation in public health spending: Correlates and consequences. *Health Serv Res.* 2009;44(5 Pt 2):1796–1817.

34. Powell C. Health departments merge Saturday: Summit County official says Akron residents will have same access to services. *Akron Beacon Journal,* December 30, 2010. http://www.ohio.com/. Accessed May 26, 2012.

35. Centers for Disease Control and Prevention. Biological and chemical terrorism: Strategic plan for preparedness and response. *MMWR.* 2000;49(RR04):1–14.

36. Centers for Disease Control and Prevention. *Public Health Preparedness: Strengthening CDC's Emergency Response (a Report on Terrorism Preparedness and Emergency Response [TPER]—Funded Activities for Fiscal Year 2007).* Atlanta: CDC; 2009.

37. National Association of County and City Health Officials. Indicators of progress in local public health preparedness. May 2008. http://www.naccho.org/publications/emergency/. Accessed May 25, 2011

38. National Association of County and City Health Officials. *Local Health Department Job Losses and Program Cuts: Findings from the January 2012 Survey.* Washington, DC: NACCHO; May 2012.

39. National Association of County and City Health Officials. *Local Health*

Department Job Losses and Program Cuts: 2008–2010. Washington, DC: NACCHO; March 2011.

40. Association of State and Territorial Health Officials. *Budget Cuts Continue to Affect the Health of Americans: Update March 2012.* Research brief. Washington, DC: ASTHO; March 2012. http://www.astho.org/Display/AssetDisplay.aspx?id=6907. Accessed May 26, 2012.

41. Association of State and Territorial Health Officials. Cuts to essential public health services jeopardize Americans' health. Press release. April 6, 2011. http://www/astho.org/t/article.aspx?artid=5839. Accessed May 25, 2011.

42. Van Wave TW, Scutchfield FD, Honore PA. Recent advances in public health systems research in the United States. *Annu Rev Public Health.* 2010;31:383–395.

43. Institute of Medicine, Committee on Public Health Strategies to Improve Health. *For the Public's Health: The Role of Measurement in Action and Accountability.* Washington, DC: National Academies Press; 2011.

44. Institute of Medicine, Committee on Public Health Strategies to Improve Health. *For the Public's Health: Revitalizing Law and Policy to Meet New Challenges.* Washington, DC: National Academies Press; 2011.

45. Institute of Medicine, Committee on Public Health Strategies to Improve Health. *For the Public's Health: Investing in a Healthier Future.* Washington, DC: National Academies Press; 2012.

46. Council on Linkages between Public Health Academia and Practice. Public Health Systems Research. http://www.phf.org/programs/council/Pages/Public_Health_SystemsResearch.aspx. Accessed June 15, 2011.

47. Fielding JE. To improve health, don't follow the money. *Am J Prev Med.* 2011;40(1 Suppl 1):S78–S79.

48. Miller W, Simon P, Maleque S, eds. *Beyond Health Care: New Directions for a Healthier America.* Washington, DC: Robert Wood Johnson Foundation Commission to Build a Healthier America; 2009.

49. Centers for Disease Control and Prevention. *National Prevention Strategy: America's Plan for Better Health and Wellness.* Atlanta: CDC; June 2011. http://www.cdc.gov/Features/PreventionStrategy/?s_cid=tw_cdc627. Accessed June 16, 2011.

50. Shaikh AR, Das IP, Vinson CA, Spring B. Cyberinfrastructure for consumer health. *Am J Prev Med.* 2011;40(1 Suppl 2):S91–S96.

51. Department of Health and Human Services. *Coordinated Federal Health Information Technology Strategic Plan: 2008–2012.* Office of the National Coordinator for Health IT. Washington, DC: DHHS; 2008.

52. Keck CW, Scutchfield FD. The future of public health. In: Scutchfield FD, Keck CW, eds. *Principles of Public Health Practice.* 3rd ed. Clifton Park, NY: Delmar Cengage Learning; 2009.

53. Bhandari MV, Scutchfield FD, Charnigo R, Riddel MC, Mays GP. New data, same story? Revisiting studies on the relationship of local public health systems characteristics to public health performance. *J Public Health Manage Pract.* 2010;16(2):110–117.

54. Lloyd P. Management in health for all: New public settings. *J Health Admin Ed.* 1994;12(2):187–207.

55. Scutchfield FD, Howard AF. Moving on upstream: The role of health

departments in addressing socioecologic determinants of disease. *Am J Prev Med.* 2011;40(1 Suppl 1):S80–S83.

56. Woolf SH, Dekker MM, Byrne FR, Miller WD. Citizen-centered health promotion: Building collaborations to facilitate healthy living. *Am J Prev Med.* 2011;40(1 Suppl 1):S38–S47.

57. Austen BioInnovation Institute in Akron. Austen BioInnovation Institute in Akron begins work on roadmap for first U.S. accountable care community. June 22, 2011. http://www.abiakron.org/austen-bioinnovation-institute-in-akron-begins-work-on-roadmap-for-first-us-accountable-care-community. Accessed July 15, 2011.

58. Cole BL, Fielding JE. Health impact assessment: A tool to help policy makers understand health beyond health care. *Annu Rev Public Health.* 2007;28:393–412.

59. Cole BL, Shimkhada R, Fielding JE, Kominski G, Morgenstern H. Methodologies for realizing the potential of health impact assessment. *Am J Prev Med.* 2005;28(4):382–389.

Contributors

Kaye Bender, PhD, RN, FAAN, is president and CEO of the Public Health Accreditation Board. She currently serves as chair of the American Public Health Association's Education Board and is past chair of the Public Health Leadership Society. She spent more than twenty years with the Mississippi State Department of Health, including five years as the deputy state health officer. She also served as dean of the University of Mississippi School of Nursing. Dr. Scutchfield is a member of the Public Health Accreditation Board.

Kevin T. Brady, MPH, is a health scientist at the Centers for Disease Control and Prevention and is the associate director for programs at the CDC Foundation in Atlanta.

Paula Braveman, MD, MPH, is director of the Center on Social Disparities in Health and professor of family and community medicine at the School of Medicine, University of California–San Francisco. Dr. Braveman focuses on documenting and understanding socioeconomic and racial or ethnic disparities in health, particularly maternal and infant health. Dr. Scutchfield has long admired her pioneering work on the social determinants of health.

Julia F. Costich, JD, PhD, is professor and associate chair of the Department of Health Services Management at the University of Kentucky College of Public Health. She served as department chair from 2005 to 2012 and was director of graduate studies for the master's of health administration degree program from 2010 to 2012. Before joining the faculty she practiced law in the public and private sectors and administered clinical programs. Dr. Scutchfield was responsible for Dr. Costich's first academic appointment in the Center for Healthcare Management and Research, a precursor of the University of Kentucky College of Public Health.

Connie J. Evashwick, ScD, FACHE, CPH, CAE, works at the nexus of health care delivery systems and public health. She was formerly the senior director of academic programs for the Association of Schools of Public Health. She has also held positions at federal, state, and local health departments; two major regional health care delivery systems; and four universities. Dr. Evashwick has been a colleague of Dr. Scutchfield's since their days in California in the 1980s; more recently they collaborated on work pertaining to hospital community benefit programming.

Paul K. Halverson, DrPH, MHSA, FACHE, is director of the Arkansas Department of Health and the state health officer, as well as the executive officer of the Arkansas State Board of Health. He is a past president of the Association of State and Territorial Health Officials. Dr. Halverson served for nearly seven years as a member of the Senior Biomedical Research Service at the Centers for Disease Control and Prevention in Atlanta. Drs. Scutchfield and Halverson worked together on developing the National Public Health Performance Standards Program, and both serve on the Public Health Accreditation Board.

Rachel Hogg, MA, is a DrPH student in health services management at the University of Kentucky College of Public Health and currently serves as a research assistant for the Center for Public Health Services and Systems Research.

James W. Holsinger Jr., MD, PhD, holds the Charles T. Wethington Jr. Endowed Chair in the Health Sciences and serves as professor of preventive medicine and health services management at the University of Kentucky College of Public Health. He previously served as undersecretary of health in the U.S. Department of Veterans Affairs (1990–1993), chancellor of the University of Kentucky Medical Center (1994–2003), and Kentucky secretary for health and family services (2003–2005). Drs. Scutchfield and Holsinger are jointly responsible for the creation of the University of Kentucky College of Public Health.

Richard Ingram, DrPH, MEd, is a research assistant professor at the University of Kentucky College of Public Health. He received his doctor of public health degree in 2010 and has been mentored by Dr. Scutchfield, serving as a graduate assistant and postdoctoral fellow in his research programs.

C. William Keck, MD, MPH, is professor emeritus and past chair of the Department of Family and Community Medicine at the Northeastern Ohio Medical University and former director of health for the city of Akron. He is past president of the American Public Health Association, the Council on Education for Public Health, the Ohio Public Health Association, the Association of Ohio Health Commissioners, and the Summit County Medical Society;

he currently chairs the Council on Linkages between Academia and Public Health Practice. Drs. Keck and Scutchfield have been close friends for forty years and are the coeditors of *Principles of Public Health Practice.*

Samuel C. Matheny, MD, MPH, holds the Nicholas Pisacano Endowed Chair and is professor of family medicine at the University of Kentucky, Department of Family and Community Medicine. He is a graduate of the University of Kentucky College of Medicine, Lexington, Kentucky, where he and Dr. Scutchfield were students together. Their careers have followed similar tracks, including employment in the U.S. Public Health Service.

David Mathews, PhD, is president of the Charles F. Kettering Foundation. He served as secretary of the Department of Health, Education, and Welfare in the Ford administration. Between 1969 and 1980 he was president of the University of Alabama. He serves on the board of a variety of organizations, including the Gerald R. Ford Foundation and the National Issues Forums Institute. Dr. Scutchfield served as a member of the faculty and associate dean of the College of Community Health Sciences at the University of Alabama during Dr. Mathews's tenure as president, and he was hosted by the Kettering Foundation during his most recent sabbatical.

W. Ryan Maynard, MBA, is a graduate of the University of Louisville and Indiana University and is a research assistant with Dr. Stephen W. Wyatt.

Glen P. Mays, PhD, MPH, is the inaugural F. Douglas Scutchfield Endowed Professor of Health Services and Systems Research at the University of Kentucky College of Public Health. Before joining the University of Kentucky in August 2011, he served as professor and chairman of the Department of Health Policy and Management in the Fay W. Boozman College of Public Health at the University of Arkansas for Medical Sciences, where he also directed the PhD program in health systems research. Drs. Mays and Scutchfield are cofounders of the field of public health services and systems research and have published extensively together.

Robin Osborn, MBA, is vice president and director of the Commonwealth Fund's International Program in Health Policy and Innovation. She is responsible for the fund's annual International Symposium on Health Policy, international health policy surveys and comparative health systems data, International Working Group on Quality Indicators, Harkness Fellowships in Health Care Policy and Practice, and international partnerships. Prior to joining the Commonwealth Fund in 1997, she directed fellowship programs at the Association for Health Services Research.

Kevin Patrick, MD, MS, is professor of family and preventive medicine at the University of California at San Diego, editor in chief of the *American Journal of Preventive Medicine,* and director of the Center for Wireless and Population Health Systems, Calit2. He is a senior adviser to the Robert Wood Johnson Foundation's Active Living Research program and a member of the National Advisory Committee of the foundation's Health Games Research initiative. He has served on the Secretary's Council for Health Promotion and Disease Prevention of the U.S. Department of Health and Human Services and on the Armed Forces Epidemiological Board. Working together, Drs. Scutchfield and Patrick and Charlotte Seidman have taken the *American Journal of Preventive Medicine* to its current level of excellence.

Debra Joy Pérez, MA, MPA, PhD, is assistant vice president for research and evaluation at the Robert Wood Johnson Foundation. In her previous capacity as a senior program officer at the foundation, much of her work focused on supporting historically underrepresented scholars through the Human Capital Team's New Connections program. Dr. Pérez is nationally recognized for building the field of public health services and systems research (PHSSR) and for developing public health practice-based research networks. She served as Dr. Scutchfield's project officer during the development of the field of PHSSR.

William J. Riley, PhD, is associate professor and associate dean at the University of Minnesota School of Public Health. He specializes in quality improvement, quality control, and safety, and his research focuses on health care administration, management, and finance. As a senior health care executive at several health care organizations, Dr. Riley has developed effective quality control systems and has led numerous process improvement initiatives. He is also the author of many studies and articles related to quality control, patient safety, and health care management and has consulted nationally on quality improvement projects.

Stephen C. Schoenbaum, MD, MPH, is special adviser to the president of the Josiah Macy Jr. Foundation. From 2000 to 2010 he was executive vice president for programs at the Commonwealth Fund and executive director of its Commission on a High Performance Health System. Prior to that, he was the medical director and later president of Harvard Pilgrim Health Care of New

England, a mixed-model HMO delivery system in Providence, Rhode Island. He is also a lecturer in the Department of Population Medicine at Harvard Medical School, a department he helped found. Drs. Scutchfield and Schoenbaum first met at the Centers for Disease Control in Atlanta in 1967, when they became Epidemic Intelligence Service officers, and they have continued their close association.

F. Douglas Scutchfield, MD, holds the Peter P. Bosomworth Endowed Professorship in Health Services Research and Policy and serves as professor of preventive medicine and health services management at the University of Kentucky College of Public Health. He was the founding director of both the Graduate School of Public Health at San Diego State University (1979–1997) and the School of Public Health at the University of Kentucky (1998–2003), now the College of Public Health. He currently directs several national centers of excellence for the Robert Wood Johnson Foundation and the Centers for Disease Control and Prevention.

Charlotte S. Seidman, FNP, MHS, MPH, ELS, is managing editor of the *American Journal of Preventive Medicine*. She graduated in the first MPH class at the Graduate School of Public Health at San Diego State University, where Dr. Scutchfield was the founding dean. She also teaches an online class on writing, editing, and peer-reviewing scientific papers for publication.

William M. Silberg, BS, is director of communications at PCORI in Washington, DC. He is the former editor at large of the *American Journal of Preventive Medicine,* where he was responsible for digital development and strategic collaborations. He is also a senior fellow at the Hunter College/CUNY Center for Health, Media, and Policy and has his own publishing and communications consulting firm. He and Dr. Scutchfield have been close associates in a variety of settings dating from their service with the American Medical Association and Medscape.

David Squires, MA, is a senior research associate in the International Program in Health Policy and Innovation at the Commonwealth Fund. His responsibilities include providing research support for the fund's annual international health policy surveys, researching and tracking health care policy developments in industrialized countries, and monitoring the research projects of the Harkness Fellows and tracking their impact on U.S. and home country health policy. Prior to joining the Commonwealth Fund, Squires worked for Abt Associates Inc. as an associate analyst in domestic health.

Steven H. Woolf, MD, MPH, is director of the Center on Human Needs at Virginia Commonwealth University and is a professor in the Department of Family Medicine. He has served as science adviser, member, and senior adviser to the U.S. Preventive Services Task Force. He focuses on the social determinants of health by addressing poverty, education, and causes of racial and ethnic disparities to improve health status, including promoting the most effective health care services and advocating the importance of health promotion and disease prevention in public health. Dr. Scutchfield has been Dr. Woolf's friend and mentor since his preventive medicine residency in the 1980s.

Stephen W. Wyatt, DMD, MPH, is dean of the College of Public Health at the University of Kentucky. Prior to his appointment, he was a commissioned officer in the U.S. Public Health Service, retiring at the rank of captain. During his tenure at the Centers for Disease Control and Prevention, Dr. Wyatt served as director of the Division of Cancer Prevention and Control and as acting deputy director of the National Center for Chronic Disease Prevention and Health Promotion. Dr. Wyatt's research interests are related to cancer prevention and control and chronic disease prevention and health promotion. Drs. Scutchfield and Wyatt were instrumental in the development of the University of Kentucky's College of Public Health.

Index

CPSIA information can be obtained at www.ICGtesting.com
Printed in the USA
BVOW081351051012

302103BV00002B/1/P